"*The Mindfulness and Acceptance Workbook for Stress Reduction* is not a workbook on how to rid yourself of those difficult feelings that get in your way. The book brings in compassion, meaningfulness, and acceptance of the inevitable. The reader is guided to develop courage and resilience in living a valued life together with feelings of stress. A well-packed course for those who want to spend more time living a vital life and less time fighting with stress."

—**JoAnne Dahl, PhD**, professor in the department of psychology at the University of Uppsala, Sweden; licensed psychologist; psychotherapist; recognized acceptance and commitment therapy (ACT) trainer; and ACBS Fellow

T0301146

"Livheim and colleagues' new stress workbook is packed with good medicine for a stressed-out world. Although the workbook is not written for professionals, therapists and health care workers will find a host of incredible tools, worksheets, and exercises for clients recovering from the stress of acute illness or learning to live more fully with chronic illness."

—**Kelly G. Wilson, PhD**, professor of psychology at the University of Mississippi, and author of *Mindfulness for Two*

"Stress reactivity is a strong predictor of poor physical and mental health. But there is something you can do: acquire the flexibility skills that will help you to change what you can change and relate differently to the things you cannot. Authored by leading experts in stress, this clear and well-written book lays out a comprehensive, step-by-step guide for targeting each of the flexibility processes known to reduce stress. Highly recommended."

—**Steven C. Hayes, PhD**, author of *Get Out of Your Mind and Into Your Life*

"Stress can make our lives miserable, but we can turn things around. This book shows you how. It is comprehensive, evidence-based, practical, and compassionate. I will be recommending it to my clients."

—**Paul Atkins, PhD**, director of prosocial psychology and senior research fellow at the Institute for Positive Psychology and Education, Australian Catholic University

"Stress is one of the most taxing and costly threats towards mental health and a prolific, sustainable life. The tools provided in this book make the mapping of stressors in your life, including your values and what makes you thrive, both fun and meaningful. The exercises offered are presented in a way that encourages you, in a self-compassionate way, to live a successful life aligned with your own values. I would like to congratulate the future readers of this book, as well as the team of scientists, practitioners, teachers, and journalists that have cocreated this very rich book that is both evidence-based, inspiring, and almost seamless to read and use."

—**Walter Osika, MD, PhD**, associate professor in the department of clinical neuroscience at Karolinska Institutet, Stockholm, Sweden; director of the Center for Social Sustainability at Karolinska Institutet, Stockholm, Sweden; and senior advisor at Stress Clinic Stockholm

The
Mindfulness & Acceptance Workbook for Stress Reduction

Using Acceptance & Commitment Therapy to Manage
Stress, Build Resilience & Create the Life You Want

FREDRIK LIVHEIM, PhD

FRANK W. BOND, PhD

DANIEL EK, MS

BJÖRN SKOGGÅRD HEDENSJÖ, MS

New Harbinger Publications, Inc.

Publisher's Note

NEW HARBINGER PUBLICATIONS is a registered trademark of New Harbinger Publications, Inc.

Distributed in Canada by Raincoast Books

Copyright © 2018 by Fredrik Livheim, Daniel Ek, Björn Skoggård Hedensjö, and Frank W. Bond
New Harbinger Publications, Inc.
5674 Shattuck Avenue
Oakland, CA 94609
www.newharbinger.com

Cover design by Amy Shoup

Acquired by Elizabeth Hollis Hansen

Edited by Kristi Hein

Library of Congress Cataloging-in-Publication Data

Names: Livheim, Fredrik, author. | Bond, Frank W., author.

Title: The mindfulness and acceptance workbook for stress reduction : using acceptance and commitment therapy to manage stress, build resilience, and create the life you want / Fredrik Livheim, PhD, Frank W. Bond, PhD, Daniel Ek, MS, and Björn Skoggård Hedensjö, MS.

Description: Oakland, CA : New Harbinger Publications, 2018. | Includes bibliographical references.

Identifiers: LCCN 2018020726 (print) | LCCN 2018023483 (ebook) | ISBN 9781684031290 (PDF e-book) | ISBN 9781684031306 (ePub) | ISBN 9781684031283 (paperback)

Subjects: LCSH: Stress (Psychology) | Stress management. | Mindfulness (Psychology) | Self-care, Health. | BISAC: SELF-HELP / Stress Management. | BODY, MIND & SPIRIT / Meditation. | PSYCHOLOGY / Mental Health. | HEALTH & FITNESS / Healthy Living.

Classification: LCC BF575.S75 (ebook) | LCC BF575.S75 L528 2018 (print) | DDC 155.9/042--dc23

LC record available at https://lccn.loc.gov/2018020726

Printed in the United States of America

24   23   22

10   9   8   7   6   5   4   3   2

Fredrik: I dedicate this book to my children, Lo, Leon, and Alve.
I want to thank you for all the love we are sharing.
You are by far the best teachers in mindfulness and playfulness I have ever met.
I also want to thank you for reminding me about what's important in life.

Daniel: To life: thanks for providing me with challenges so that I can learn, friends to help me when I'm lost, parents so I can get through, and forests so that I can breathe.

Björn: This book is for my beloved mother, Kerstin, who passed away while we were writing it. Without you there would have been nothing.

Frank: To Aidan, who continually gives me the courage to "be," and to live more in accordance with myself.

Contents

Introduction

Imagine having a monkey on your shoulder chattering endlessly into your ear about what a failure you are. It might say: "You're not very productive at work, are you? And you really should start working out again. Why are you such a bore? Why can't you be more interesting?" After a brief pause, it carries on: "At least you've managed to keep your family together—but you know you did that at the expense of your career. And it's not like you're really trying to get ahead at work, either." Or maybe it says: "You're a fake and you know it—it won't be long until it's plain to everyone else as well. You'd better step up your game at work before you're found out."

For many of us, there is no need to fantasize about a malicious monkey; we already have an inner voice that frequently puts us down. This may be one reason why you picked up this book. Or maybe there's something a bit "off" in your life. Maybe you're trying to find a better balance in your life: more fun, less hassle and bother. Maybe you're wishing you had more time for the things that really matter to you: spending time with family and friends, committing to a romantic relationship, being in the moment, or just getting some well-deserved rest and relaxation. Or you could be reading this book for another reason completely. You may have a family member or a close friend who is not doing well. Perhaps you're feeling unhappy and excluded at work or in other areas of your life. Maybe you are feeling burned out by the pressure of it all. Whatever situation you find yourself in, this book will help you manage these life stresses and pains.

We will help you to do this in a way based on scientific evidence, so it is likely to work for you. Our program involves techniques that you may have heard about or even tried (such as developing problem-solving skills) and ones that may be new to you (such as how you respond to your feelings). You will quickly see that your choice of technique in a given situation may depend on which ones help you (perhaps ultimately) achieve meaning and vitality in your life. As you will see, knowing you are moving in directions you value can make even the most difficult circumstances less stressful.

A NINE-STEP PROGRAM FOR MASTERING STRESS

This program will help you:

- Understand how stress shows up in your life

- Live a more meaningful life directed by your deepest values

- Change the causes of stress that you can control

- Approach the feelings of unavoidable stress in a new way that won't sabotage your goals

- Take a mindful stance toward your difficult emotions and thoughts

- Become a better friend to yourself

- Strengthen relationships and connect better with people in general

- Accomplish things you may not even yet know you wish to do

A SCIENCE-BASED PROGRAM

The program this book describes is based on over thirty years of scientifically proven theory, strategies, and techniques. Unsurprisingly, it has an excellent track record for helping people live lives that they value and don't feel overwhelmed by. For handling stress alone, we have tested and published this program since 1997. This program is based primarily on an evidence-based psychological model called acceptance and commitment therapy (Hayes, Strosahl, & Wilson, 2012). We call it by its acronym, ACT, pronounced just like the verb. Saying it as a word underlines the importance of taking *act*-ion. The "t" in act can refer to "therapy" or "training," depending on the context in which you are using it. In the workplace, we use "training," as some workers would rather not think they are signing up for "therapy."

ACT

ACT is one of the newer forms of cognitive behavioral therapy (CBT), focused on how we can approach our thoughts, feelings, memories, and urges in ways that are more helpful to us. In this life, all seven-plus billion of us humans strive to be happy—an effort that unites us all, across all cultures and times. And we also share the reality that we do not always get what we want, we face difficulties, we mess up, we doubt ourselves, and we sometimes lose our grip. ACT is about making space for the beautiful and amazing in life, and also for its pain and sorrow. ACT assumes that it is impossible to fully control or get rid of most internal responses, such as unwanted thoughts and feelings. But we can learn to let go of our struggle against them and to live a meaningful life *together with* these thoughts and feelings, in a new way.

WHY THIS BOOK IS DIFFERENT

We want to be clear that ACT is not just another brand name for some combination of problem solving and meditation or mindfulness techniques. Mindfulness is the ability to be present, in the here and now, with openness to and curiosity about what you are experiencing in your body: your thoughts, feelings, physical sensations, memories, and urges. With ACT, you can think of mindfulness as a way of relating to these internal responses that helps you be less distressed by them. For example, if a window is open while you are comfortably reading, and you begin to hear a small buzzing sound, you may wonder if that's a fly annoying you or a wasp that could also hurt you. By responding mindfully to these sudden concerns, you would notice the concerns, the changes to your breathing, and any other discomfort you may experience. By doing so, you may be responding to these experiences very differently for the first time, instead of buying into them or being compelled by what they seem to urge you to do. Such mindful responding will probably make you feel less stressed to begin with, and it will also allow you to continue to enjoy pursuing your goal of reading.

In contrast, if you weren't mindful, you could be at the mercy of your thoughts and fears, chasing that insect all around the room until you are exhausted, frustrated, and, if it turns out to be a wasp, eventually stung! Plus, you would not have been pursuing what is actually meaningful to you at that time: relaxing while reading a book. By not being mindful, you would be in a lose-lose situation: painfully exhausted and not doing what is meaningful to you.

With ACT, mindfulness is not focused simplistically on making you more relaxed and less anxious; rather, mindfulness is a way for you to rethink your patterns and to practice carrying your difficult thoughts, feelings, memories, and urges, so that when you open your eyes, stand up, and face the real world, you can move toward your goals more effectively. As readers of other mindfulness books may already be seeing, the ACT emphasis is on taking action, with the *help* of mindfulness.

Now, here's a good question: does ACT even work? Of course it does, or we wouldn't have taken the time to write this book! In fact, there are about fourteen "gold standard" studies showing that ACT can help us reduce stress, depression, and anxiety (see, for example, Frögéli et al., 2016; Lloyd, Bond, & Flaxman, 2013; Flaxman & Bond, 2010a; Flaxman & Bond, 2010b; Livheim et al., 2015; Brinkborg, Michanek, Hesser, & Berglund, 2011; Bond & Bunce, 2000). One of these studies even used ACT as an online self-help tool, and research showed this led to very favorable long-term improvements in reducing stress and improving life quality, as measured up to one year after completion of the training (Räsänen, Lappalainen, Muotka, Tolvanen, & Lappalainen, 2016). A new study (French, Golijani-Moghaddama, & Schröder, in press), which summarizes all studies of ACT practiced by using self-help books or Internet resources, states that ACT self-help is an effective intervention. And a study of ACT self-help in book format specifically for reducing stress shows that reading an ACT book, without any contact with a therapist, provided significant stress reduction and decreased symptoms of burnout (Hofer et al., in press).

Unlike many other life-enhancing approaches, ACT accepts theories and research findings that show we cannot consistently, sufficiently, and reliably get rid of our difficult thoughts or feelings without resorting to harmful methods (such as taking drugs). So instead of trying to relive our lives to find the love we didn't experience as children, perhaps ACT can show us how to approach that pain so that we can devise a way to connect with and love people, beginning now.

Here's a thought: Even if we could magically relive our lives and erase painful experiences, wouldn't we also lose key parts of our history and experiences that make us who we uniquely are? Thus, perhaps we are too ready to be rid of our difficult thoughts and feelings. It may be more useful to think of them as medals that you have earned bys living your life. They represent your humanity, and they allow you to more easily connect with those other humans who are traveling parts of the same path that you are, finding meaning and vitality. So, far from trying to get rid of them, wear your medals of difficult thoughts and feelings with the knowledge that they can help you connect with other humans along your journey (which may also make your trip through life a bit more interesting).

In addition to teaching you mindfulness skills, we will lead you, step by step, through how to face difficult emotions and, where possible, to transform life hassles that get you stuck. Throughout the book we will use the technique of mindfulness as the key stance to adopt in your life, to realize the meaningful life that you seek.

Authors Fredrik Livheim and Daniel Ek are licensed psychologists with professional experience in stress management, focused on the prevention and treatment of negative stress and burnout syndrome; Björn Skoggård Hedensjö is a science reporter and clinical psychologist; and Frank W. Bond is professor of psychology and management and has conducted research in the ACT field, particularly in areas of performance and mental health. Speaking as both therapists and scientists, we aimed to give you an easy-to-read guide of the best advice that we, and the rest of the scientific community, can offer you to live a vital and manageable life. We have had independent reviewers, including brain researchers, fact-check this book to verify that its content is in line with the latest science.

This book is designed as a manageable self-help program stretching over nine weeks, with a new step each week. When you've finished the book, you will have a better understanding of how stress shows up in your life, and you will have taken new steps to handle challenges in more skillful ways. You will also have gained tools to live a more meaningful life and to boost your well-being. We are confident that by using the skills in this book you can end up in a better place, with a more well-balanced life. Based on the data and our experiences in introducing ACT to thousands of stressed people, the odds are in your favor!

HOW TO USE THIS BOOK

You can use this book on its own or as a complement to any type of counseling or therapy that you may be undertaking. Alternatively, you could form a study group or read it more informally with friends (why not form a book club?). Each of the nine chapters has a core section and an expanded section. We suggest that you read one chapter a week, actively trying to make use of the advice and the exercises that we recommend throughout that week. There is no need to rush through the book. The greatest possible benefit comes from digesting the book at your own pace and turning our advice, and your own experience, into concrete behaviors that lead you to experience a better life, day after day. There are also a host of materials available for download at the website for this book: http://www .newharbinger.com/41283. (See the very back of this book for more details.)

In addition to the advice and information provided in each chapter, we will also discuss the lives of "John" and "Angela," two composite, representative people we have created from working with clients. They are people you may be able to relate to in some way, having typical difficulties coping with stress in their daily lives. We hope that by exploring their experiences and seeing how they cope with their everyday problems, you'll recognize some challenges you face, too, and be inspired to come up with your own solutions.

How This Book Is Structured

Chapters 1 through 8 each start with a core section followed by an expanded section.

CORE SECTION

If you're stressed out, pressed for time, or don't like reading very much, you'll find these key principles for understanding and coping with stress in the core section:

- Information on stress and the basic principles for striking a better balance in life

- Exercises that can help you understand your stress and choose the recovery methods that suit you best

- Advice to try out for the following week

EXPANDED SECTION

If you want in-depth information on what you've just read in the core section, we recommend that you read the expanded section, where we offer more exercises and knowledge to aid in your journey toward challenging unhealthy habits and taking control of your life. The expanded section also contains science sections with relevant findings from the fields of brain research and neuropsychology (the study of how the function of the brain relates to psychological behaviors). These were written by Pär Flodin, a researcher in brain imaging and cognitive neuroscience at Karolinska Institutet.

We believe you will benefit the most from this book by reading the expanded sections as well as the core sections. But if you choose to skip the expanded sections, that's perfectly okay. Just focus on practicing what you've learned from the core sections in your daily life.

We recommend that you try out the advice in this book as much as possible. Give our recommendations a fair chance; some that you may find silly at first could turn out to be the ones that help you the most! Also, try not to be afraid to take a chance on a technique, even if you occasionally come across recommendations that you are unfamiliar with or don't think will really work for you; you may be pleasantly surprised! We recommend that you carry this book with you while you are going through it, in your handbag, backpack, or briefcase. That way, you will always have exercises and advice close at hand whenever you need them. It will also remind you that we—and our years of research—are here with you on this exciting and challenging journey to make your life as vital as possible.

The First Step Toward
a Less Stressful Life

It is not stress that kills us but our reaction to it.

—Hans Selye

You're late for the bus, and you just manage to squeeze in through the doors before they close. What you didn't miss, however, was the big muddy puddle on the sidewalk as you dashed for the bus. Now your trousers are splattered with mud. Your mind starts racing. "I'm such a klutz. Why does this always have to happen to me? How will my boss react when I walk into the meeting with a new client looking like a bum?" Yesterday, your boss stressed more than once how important this meeting was for the future of the company. You suddenly feel intense stomach pain. Then your mind drifts to all the things you have to do that afternoon. Oh, and don't forget that you're a failure as a parent, too: you'll probably be the last parent to pick up your kid at kindergarten—again.

You try to clear your mind by checking emails on your phone. Twelve new messages, and you haven't even reached the office yet! How will you ever find the time to read and reply to them all? Your heart starts racing, and you break into a cold sweat.

Does this sound familiar? Even if the start of your day wasn't quite as bad as this, you most likely recognized some aspects of it from your own life.

In this scenario, you experience something we all suffer from at least every now and then: a stress reaction.

CORE SECTION: HOW STRESS WORKS

The stress reaction is our response to a challenge. It's a primordial and life-saving response that mobilizes both body and mind. Without stress, we would probably become passive, depressed, and unproductive. What we call short-term stress is actually quite beneficial: it helps us focus and get things done. The problem with stress is that, without recovery, short-term stress can turn into long-term chronic stress, which can in turn lead to negative and serious psychological and physical symptoms (Savic, Perski, & Osika, in press; Hains et al., 2009; Arnsten, 2009). For example, with long-term stress, the body's ability to fight infections is significantly lowered, so we are more prone to catch contagious diseases. Also, the stress hormone cortisol stays at high levels and can adversely affect our memory functions (Liston, McEwen, & Casey, 2009; Klingberg, 2009). Over time, chronic stress can lead to, among other things, intestinal problems, obesity, increases in blood pressure, sleeping problems, and depression (Piazza et al., 2013; Segerstrom & Miller, 2004; Radley et al., 2006).

Figure 1 clearly and concisely depicts the effects of long-term chronic stress. The gray upper curve shows how the normal stress level rises if there is no recovery or recharging. The black curve below it illustrates the importance of rest and recharge. If we allow ourselves regular periods of rest and recharge, our normal stress is unlikely to rise to a harmful level.

A stress reaction often occurs when you feel that the demands you are facing exceed your perceived ability to cope with them. Many demands contribute to stress and chronic stress (Bakker & Demerouti, 2007). Sometimes the demands within a certain period of your life may feel like too much to handle. Other times, the sum of all the (perhaps small) demands from many different areas of your life may combine to simply overwhelm you. In these cases, you may neglect friendships, exercise, or sleep so you can deal with all the things (real or imagined) you feel obligated to do. This serves only to increase your stress, though—and this is when it can become chronic and harmful.

What causes stress is somewhat individual, of course, but there are situations that can cause stress in almost anyone, particularly:

- Situations that are new and unfamiliar

- Situations where you don't have the complete picture and the outcome is hard to predict

- Situations where you feel little control or influence

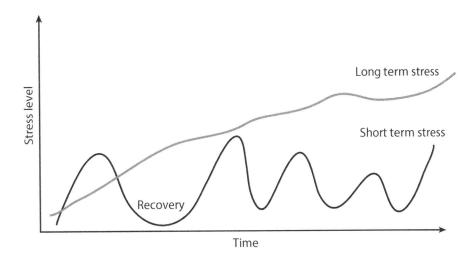

Figure 1: The difference between short-term and long-term stress

Common examples of situational stress are being fired, getting diagnosed with a chronic illness, going through a divorce, and becoming a parent. But it can also be something less obviously stressful, like having to prepare a speech at work on a subject in which you lack experience.

We've compiled a list of demands and situations that many people find stressful, especially if they occur at the same time. Do you recognize any of these in your life right now? Circle the ones you are currently experiencing.

Death in the family

Relationship problems, breakups, divorce

Being harassed or ostracized at work

Illness—your own or a family member's

Becoming a parent

Mental health issues

Physical problems

Sexual difficulties

Heavy workload

Complex assignments

Trouble with boss

Restructuring at work

Problems with family or friends

Moving to a new home

Facing financial difficulties (including major mortgage)

A family member in distress

Child leaving home

Feeling a lack of control

Job interviews

Not enough hours in the day

A new job

Meeting an impossible deadline

Does your list of personal stress triggers include some not on this list? Take a minute and write down the demands you face in your life right now: your own examples from the list, and perhaps others that are not listed. Don't hold back! We will return to them later.

Stressful Things I'm Experiencing Right Now:

_____

_____

_____

_____

Typical Signs of Stress

There are four categories of stress symptoms: physical sensations (body), thinking (mind-set), emotions (mood), and actions (behavior). It is typical to have symptoms in more than one of these categories. The following lists present the categories of common stress symptoms; check all that apply to you. If you don't see symptoms that you normally experience, write them on the lines that follow.

Body (Physical Symptoms)	Mind-set
Sleeping problems	Confusion
Headaches	Alienation, detachment
Stomachaches	Difficulty letting go of work
Palpitations	Difficulty prioritizing
Muscle tension	Difficulty concentrating
Pain	Forgetfulness
Dry mouth	Tunnel vision, limited view
Impotence/low libido	
Dizziness	
Jumpiness, clumsiness	

Mood

Anxious, worried

Guilt-ridden, ashamed

Emotionally drained

Sad

Irritated, angry

Exhausted

Subject to tears

Devoid of feeling, numb

Behavior

Strives for efficiency

Is always in a hurry

Stops taking breaks

Eats too fast

Walks around aimlessly

Does things twice

Is controlling, obsessed with details

Stops listening to others

Argumentative and irritable, swears a lot

Copes by using alcohol or drugs

Eats much more or less than normal

Body:

_____

_____

_____

_____

_____

Mind-set:

_____

_____

_____

_____

_____

Mood:

_____

_____

_____

_____

_____

Behavior:

_____

_____

_____

_____

_____

The Stress Spiral to Sickness

Stress responses originally evolved to be beneficial to humans. When we were roaming the African savannah, our stress responses allowed us to eat dinner instead of being the dinner eaten. Clearly, few people today normally face such life-or-death situations in their daily lives. Stress can still provide the house warrior in us with the adrenaline and attentional focus we need to get the kids off to school. It can help us to simultaneously notice that the baby is being too curious about the sharp knife we accidentally left on the table while we are trying to get another kid's arm into his coat sleeve.

The problem with stress today is not that it occurs, as it can be useful to give us focus, energy, and attention. The problem arises when it goes on for too long and begins to grow increasingly strong, a gravitational pull that drags your whole body and ability to function properly down into a hole. Let's see how this cruel stress spiral can begin to build:

Situation

Something happens in your life that makes you feel anxious. It could be a new and unpredictable situation where you experience a lack of control: someone falls ill, you go through a breakup, you get swamped with work, or you start a new job. Sometimes, the accumulation of small changes is what triggers a stress response.

Urgency/Responsibility/Importance

Maybe you feel that the stressor is solely or largely your responsibility, that the issue is very important and urgent, and that you cannot and must not fail. This can lead you to feel even more stressed out, anxious, and tense all over.

Extra Effort/Neglecting Needs

You feel an urge to immediately resolve the matter at hand; you mobilize to actively try to solve the problem. You go the extra mile, you work overtime, and if someone else is a bit under the weather, you try to be there for them to help out. To make time for this, you neglect doing the things that normally help you recuperate, such as spending time with friends, working out, or sleeping properly.

Payoff/Reward

That final push ultimately pays off. You get rewarded somehow. Maybe people around you feel better; your boss, colleagues, or you yourself feel you accomplished your task or responsibility. You resolved some of the issues that have been stressing you out—for the moment. Your anxiety and tension levels are slightly lowered, but there is still a lurking fear that this process can all start again at any time—perhaps because it often does.

Reinforcement of Extra Effort/Neglecting Needs

By successfully responding to the initial stressful situation, you have rewarded and reinforced a behavior where you always resolve a difficult situation by taking responsibility, putting in extra work, and neglecting recovery, thereby increasing the likelihood of repeating a negative pattern. You'll keep rolling up your sleeves, taking on the role of Mr. or Ms. Fix-It. But you pay a price: less recovery time, and increasingly chronic stress. Simply put, your mind and your actions are writing checks your body can't cash.

Example: Angela's Stress Spiral

At the end of the chapter you will meet Angela in more detail. This is her stress spiral.

Situation

My daughter is going through a difficult divorce.
There is a lot of pressure at work.

↓

Urgency/Responsibility/Importance

My daughter needs me. I cannot let her down. I need to
be there for her. I cannot fail my colleagues; we're a team.

↓

Extra Effort/Neglecting Needs

I make sure my daughter has everything she needs. I help her
out with the chores at her home. I take time to listen to her.
I take on more tasks at work and make the extra effort
for my colleagues.

↓

Payoff/Reward

My daughter's burdens are lessened. She expresses great
appreciation for my help; she says she couldn't cope without
me. I feel that I am a great help to her; I feel less worried.

At work, my colleagues also express appreciation for my
efforts. I feel useful and helpful.

↓

Reinforcement of Extra Effort/Neglecting Needs

Angela keeps on going the extra mile for her daughter and
colleagues at work. She runs faster just to stay in one place,
until she can no longer keep up that pace. At that point,
something has to give.

EXERCISE: YOUR STRESS SPIRAL

If you have some idea of what could be starting and building up your stress cycle, you might be able to intervene before you go down into that hole. In the following boxes, think about the last time you experienced a stress cycle, and, using Angela's example, fill in the boxes. Notice that you can intervene to slow or stop this cycle by doing something in at least one of the boxes (for example, change your situation briefly by taking a nap).

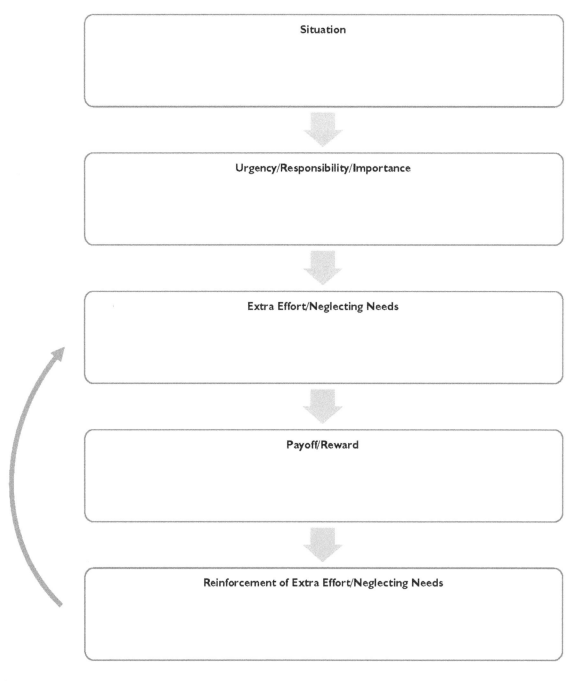

Check Your Stress Levels

Of course, an ounce of prevention is worth a pound of cure, so let's have a look at your current stress levels. They may be fine; they may be getting a bit high, so you want to start thinking about where in the cycle to intervene; or they may be very high, so you need to do something *now*! Let's not prejudge your situation yet, though. Our scientific scale can help with that!

The Perceived Stress Scale is one of the most widely used psychological instruments for measuring how stressed out you're feeling (e.g., Cohen & Janicki-Deverts, 2012). There are no "right" or "wrong" answers to the questions (so you can be honest!), so don't spend too much time thinking about each item; just circle the number for the response that seems to sum up your overall experience over the last month. You will get an opportunity to complete this again later on in the book to see how you are coming along.

In the last month, how often have you ...	Never	Almost never	Sometimes	Fairly often	Very often
... been upset because of something that happened unexpectedly?	0	1	2	3	4
... felt that you were unable to control the important things in your life?	0	1	2	3	4
... felt nervous and stressed?	0	1	2	3	4
... felt confident about your ability to handle your personal problems?	4	3	2	1	0
... felt that things were going your way?	4	3	2	1	0
... found that you could not cope with all the things that you had to do?	0	1	2	3	4
... been able to control irritations in your life?	4	3	2	1	0
... felt that you were on top of things?	4	3	2	1	0
... been angered because of things that were outside of your control?	0	1	2	3	4
... felt difficulties were piling up so high that you could not overcome them?	0	1	2	3	4

Interpreting Your Answers

You're the expert on you. Only you can tell how stressed out you really are. But if you like, you can compare your score to those of thousands of others (Chan & La Greca, 2013) who have taken this test to determine what category you may fall into: low, average, or high stress. Start by just adding up your scores. If your score is anywhere from 0 to 7, your stress level is rather low—stress is not a big problem for you right now. Still, you might find this book helpful in preventing future problems, and minimizing those that you have. If your score is from 8 to 20, you probably have moderate stress problems in your daily life—you definitely have issues to work on. We recommend that you read and follow the advice in this book. If your score is 20 or higher, you are most likely suffering from serious stress problems and would probably benefit greatly from reading and following the advice in this book. You may also wish to consult a professional, such as your general practitioner or a therapist.

We've now covered the basics: what stress is, how it works, and your stress profile. Now we invite you to explore what you really want out of life and to identify what brings it purpose and vitality. Clearly this is important anyway, but knowing you are working toward those values, even using baby steps, can help you manage your stress.

EXERCISE: ARE YOU LIVING THE LIFE YOU WANT?

Throughout the book, you will have opportunities to explore what's important to you. We'll ask you to consider making even small course corrections that could potentially steer you toward a more balanced life in terms of experiencing what is meaningful to you. Your life is the sum total of the things you do every day. You have only a limited number of days and hours on this earth, so you'd better make them count. Ponder the following:

Where would you be ten years from now if you were to stick to your current priorities, while ignoring others? What would your life be like then? What would you have accomplished, and what would you have missed out on? Do you feel you need to make any changes to accomplish what is most meaningful to you?

How my life would be: _____

_____

Would have accomplished: _____

_____

Would have missed out on: _____

_____

Changes I see that I would need to make to follow my values: _____

_____

Imagine making a lasting change that reduces your stress levels by setting priorities that bring you closer to doing those things and seeing those people that are important to you. How would that change where you would be in ten years' time? Would you be in good health, or even alive? What would you have accomplished that is meaningful to you, and what would you have missed out on that you value? To what degree would these changes be worth it to you (keeping in mind how much you value the feelings of anyone you may love)?

How my life would be: _____

_____

Would have accomplished: _____

_____

Would have missed out on: _____

_____

How much are the changes worth to me? _____

_____

Schedule Recharging Activities

The problem with stress is not stress itself, but the lack of proper recharging. You can think of your body and mind using the analogy of a smartphone. The phone needs energy to function; it needs to be charged, and sometimes it also needs to "rest"—to be turned off so as not to overheat. Similarly, our bodies and minds need a recharging of energy, which we may get from an intense workout, seeing a good friend, or just relaxing. We like the word "recharge," because it encompasses both active and more passive activities. Sometimes we forget to make time for recharging and rejuvenation of both body and mind. A good way to strike a better balance in life is by beginning to actually *schedule* these activities. Make it one of your top priorities. After a period of prolonged stress, it's not unusual to feel even more stressed out when trying to schedule restorative activities. It is not uncommon for stressful thoughts to pop up, such as "How will I ever make time for this?" or "I cannot prioritize a relaxing activity now!" Trying to make time for recovery can be an emotionally draining process.

Indeed, coming to terms with their actual stress levels can be an uncomfortable experience for many people. Some face emotions they had been trying to avoid, for example, by burying themselves in work. Feelings such as loneliness, sorrow, anger, and related internal responses (such as thoughts, feelings, and physiological sensations) sometime come to the surface. In the chapters that follow, we will discuss ways you can approach these types of challenging internal responses so you can more effectively recover. This is important, as scientists agree that recharging is vital to bringing about lasting change, even if you initially might feel some discomfort in trying to do so. Trust us—it will get easier with time, and so too will your success at recovery.

EXERCISE: YOUR RECHARGING ACTIVITIES

We now invite you to make a list of the activities and situations that enable you to recover, relax, and recharge. These could be things that you currently enjoy doing or things you have enjoyed in the past. Or perhaps you're thinking of things you've never done but would like to do. We've listed examples of both active and passive activities. Notice that some of these restorative activities don't take a lot of time: some can take five minutes, while others can take five days!

Leisure time

Playing a musical instrument, cuddling a pet, watching a movie or a TV series, checking out a funny video clip, listening to music or dancing, reading a book, taking a bath or a long shower, going to the movies (even by yourself), pausing for a minute or two, having a cup of coffee or tea, making room for a hobby, or having some alone time.

Relationships

Meeting a friend for a cup of coffee or tea, calling family and friends, going to the movies with a friend, texting something nice to someone you know, taking a trip with someone, treating a coworker to lunch, scheduling an activity with a friend, or making a dinner "date" with your partner.

Health

Taking a nap during the day, going for a walk, cooking one of your favorite dishes, having a nice cup of tea, going horseback riding, going to the gym, playing with a child, running, practicing mindfulness, praying or meditating, doing yoga, having sex, or getting a massage.

Work/education/volunteering

Taking short breaks at work, complimenting someone, going for a coffee or a long lunch with a coworker, going for a walk during your lunch break, walking up to a colleague and praising his or her skills, practicing mindfulness at work, going outside to breathe for five minutes, pausing for a minute or two, or focusing on one task at a time.

If you can volunteer in addition to or instead of paid employment, what interests you? Are you a political animal who follows your representatives closely? Then contributing to a related organization may help you create even more meaning from your interests.

Write down how you'd like to recover from stress:

Leisure time: _____

_____

_____

_____

_____

Relationships: _____

_____

_____

_____

_____

Health: _____

_____

_____

_____

_____

Work/education/volunteering: _____

_____

_____

_____

_____

TAKING ACTION: WHAT YOU CAN DO BEFORE READING THE NEXT CHAPTER

The purpose of this book is to empower you to make the changes necessary for achieving a healthy balance in your life—one step at a time. As you begin listing the recovery activities that you do (or would like to do) over the next two weeks, think about which ones bring you the most meaning and sense of accomplishment. These feelings of vitality may indicate that you are working toward something you value in your life.

Values will be a primary focus of the next chapter. We think of a value as the basis of actions you take—big or small—that truly mean something to you and that you keep working on, like being a good father. We have values that relate to our entire lives (such as honesty) or that are specific to one area (such as family). In every situation, though, we can choose to let our values guide our choices, considering how our behavior will reflect the values we could bring to our current situation. We can view goals and problem solving as plans to ensure that we work toward our values and don't waste time on activities that won't be meaningful to us. Our values specify the actions that, taken together, serve as concrete examples of them. For example, if you value being a good father, you may have a goal to attend eight out of ten of your child's football matches. Achieving that is a sure sign that's one of your genuine values. As you will see, problem solving also can help you achieve that goal.

As you identify your recharging activities over the next two weeks, see if certain ones bring a sense of accomplishment and achievement as well as recovery. We hope you will realize that you tend to feel a sense of vitality when you take actions that reflect your values. This can help you overcome the pain of stress. So this week's assignment is important because you'll explore activities in different areas of your life that you may value. Once you get a sense of these, you'll learn how to manage the fears and difficult internal and external events that may get in the way of your working toward your values, and you'll begin to loosen that noose of stress around your neck.

We suggest you do the following in the coming week:

Read the next chapter. Schedule a day for reading Chapter 2 of this book. About a week from now would be ideal. Make a note in your calendar or set an alarm on your phone.

Recharge. Pick one to three recovering activities for the coming week and put them in your calendar. Schedule a time and a place for these activities, and arrange a time to do one with a friend, if appropriate. Set an alarm on your phone if you find that helpful. If any distressing thoughts arise during these activities, simply note them and bring them along on your activity.

FOLLOW JOHN AND ANGELA IN THEIR EFFORTS TO LIVE A MORE MEANINGFUL AND BALANCED LIFE

Throughout this book, you will be able to follow these two people who have used the strategies in this book on their journeys to a more meaningful and balanced life. We each have our own unique life situation, so your thoughts and answers will, of course, differ from theirs. That's okay; see what you can learn from their experiences.

John

Hello, my name is John, and I'm thirty-four years old. These last two years have been pretty rough. I work in a research and development (R&D) department for environmental control systems in various fields. I actually find this job stimulating, and I feel as if I've finally found what I'm good at. Unfortunately, the company is struggling to make ends meet, and I've had to work a lot of overtime lately. When I started this job, my relationship ended. My partner and I were very close, and we did everything as a couple. I wasn't completely heartbroken by it, but on the other hand, I do have a tendency to numb myself with work. Somehow I've ended up in a place where I have no time for my friends or myself. I manage to work out quite a bit, but other than that, I don't do much outside of work.

Things that trigger my stress symptoms:

Job demands—learning new systems

Breakup with partner

Swamped with work

Behavior and stress symptoms:

Not sleeping well; waking up early, not fully rested

Muscle tension and cramping

Shallow breathing

Irritability

Feeling low

Plan for reading Chapter 2 of this book:

I have some spare time next Sunday after dinner.

My recharging activities for next week and what reminders to use:

■ See if Ethan or Mary wants to go out to dinner on Friday night.

■ Work out on Tuesday at 5 p.m. (even if I'm not completely done at work).

■ I've set an alarm on my smartphone as a reminder.

Angela

Hello, my name is Angela, and I'm fifty years old. I've worked in teaching and caring professions all of my life. I was a kindergarten teacher for quite some time, but right now I'm working as a nursing assistant. Working with people can be exhausting. I rarely take time to meet with friends or other people after work. The fact that everyone else is stressed out during coffee breaks is not exactly helpful either. If we even get to take breaks! My husband says I should slow down and stop covering for everyone else. He thinks I have a hard time saying no. I always do my best—I never want anyone to say that I'm not pulling my weight. But to some extent I guess he's right. I've started to notice how I never seem to have enough energy. I feel empty inside, and my work isn't fun anymore. I used to be an early riser and the first one to arrive at work. Heck, I even had energy to spare; back then, I would put everyone's dishes in the dishwasher before I went to work. Nowadays, I spend my week longing for the weekend. Come Sunday evening, I feel uneasy and tense. My daughter just got divorced, and I think that has added some extra weight on my shoulders as well.

Things that trigger my stress symptoms:

Saying no to people at work

Overachieving at work

Thoughts about needing to do more, to keep busy

"Needing" to skip breaks at work

My daughter's divorce

Behavior and stress symptoms:

Not doing things that I enjoy

Giving extra time to my daughter; I feel I am responsible to make her feel better

Neglecting my friends

Having occasional panic attacks and trouble breathing

Sleeping a lot

Plan for reading Chapter 2 of this book:

I plan to read Chapter 2 on Thursday night. The expanded section in Chapter 1 was interesting to read, so I think I'll read the expanded section for Chapter 2 as well.

My recovering activities for next week and what reminders to use:

■ After work on Tuesday, I've planned a walk in the woods (the same route I used to take years ago). Call Christina to see if she wants to tag along!

■ Ask hubby if he wants to watch a movie at home on Saturday night, complete with snacks and drinks.

■ Eat properly at work! On Wednesday and Friday, I've planned to go to a restaurant I like not far from work.

■ I have noted this in my calendar and on a sticky note on the refrigerator.

You've been reading the *core section* of the chapter. You've learned the basic principles behind understanding stress and that the most important component in stress management is recovery. Would you like to learn more about stress and the inner workings of the brain? Might a tool for getting things done and staying focused be useful for you at work? More information is available in the *expanded section* that follows, so if you have the interest or time, read on! If not, we'll see you in the next chapter, and good luck with your recovering activities.

CHAPTER 1 EXPANDED SECTION

In this section you will find more exercises and additional information to help you influence and change your life situation. We'll cover short-term stress and chronic stress, how our thoughts can trigger stress, and the effects of chronic stress on the brain. We will also provide a simple tool for getting things done and staying focused. If you are interested in yet another tool for keeping track of both your stress triggers in daily life and your recharging activities, you can download the Stress and Recharge Journal at the website for this book: http://www.newharbinger.com/41283.

Stress Is Essential to Our Survival

Modern humans with linguistic capabilities have been around for at least a hundred thousand years. We've spent 99 percent of that time living in the wilderness, where we faced dangers of a very different kind than those we come across today. Back then we needed to be alert and aware of our surroundings, lest we fall victim to wild animals or rival tribes. Only people who learned to deal with danger at a young age lived on to procreate. Therefore, you could argue that everyone alive today is the result of a breeding program that has stretched over thousands of generations, rewarding the ability to react effectively to danger. If our ancestors came face to face with a dangerous animal in the wilderness, they had two choices: fighting back or trying to outrun it. This is what psychologists call a fight-or-flight response, one of our most basic stress responses.

Short-Term Stress

When the fight-or-flight response activates in a threatening situation, it gives you a temporary performance boost: body and mind are mobilized to avert the threat. The heart starts pumping faster to increase the blood flow to all major muscles and supply the body with more oxygen, and our thinking becomes almost entirely focused on survival. The purpose is to boost our body's strength and speed. This state of short-term or acute stress can be helpful to us, although it's more helpful when we are *really* under physical threat. Regardless of the kind of threat, our bodies are built to cope with such short-term stress. Short-term stress in modern life might occur in connection with an accident or when you're in a difficult situation, need to run to catch the bus, or are about to make a presentation. When the immediate danger has been averted, when you've caught the bus or finished your presentation, your body immediately starts to recover. After a while, the body has regained its balance and starts to rebuild its resources to prepare for the next challenge.

Chronic Stress: Its Symptoms and Consequences

Long-term stress, also known as chronic stress, is often less intense and not as obvious to the afflicted person as short-term stress. Chronic stress might manifest as a never-ending, grinding concern over finding the right balance between work and family life. You might see this as a natural part of life. Nevertheless, it is still stressful. As a consequence, you might have abandoned a favorite pastime because you couldn't fit it into your schedule. Or maybe you've neglected to call a friend for weeks—or months. You keep telling yourself that sometime soon there will come a time for taking walks, enjoying the scenery, or relaxing with a book—somewhere further down the road, when you're finally out of the *figurative* woods. Pausing and reflecting on your life can be very unpleasant when you're already afflicted by stress. These feelings can manifest as physical afflictions or as psychological pains such as sadness, anger, loneliness, or anxiety. But if we fail to face these feelings, to pause for a moment every now and then, we risk neglecting important natural warning signals that might otherwise help us turn our lives around and bring about real change.

When your motor is already running, it's tempting to take on the next big assignment without stopping to refuel first and reflect on whether you should take on the assignment. When at full speed, we might neglect signals of hunger, fatigue, or even the need to go to the bathroom. Again, the body displays negative and serious symptoms when suffering from chronic stress. This type of stress is detrimental to our physical health and can also bring about depression or other mental health problems.

The stress response for fight or flight is essential to our survival and actually harmless—as long as we give ourselves a chance to recover.

The Freeze Response

Another type of survival instinct, or stress response, is what psychologists call freezing behavior, freeze response, or writer's or designer's block. The body freezes, becomes passive, and even powers down its internal functions. We can lose the ability to think effectively, never mind creatively. We can see these reactions in prey animals as they try to avoid being detected by predators with good eyesight. Sometimes these animals even feign death, since most predators prefer a live prey, not a dead one. You may recognize having this reaction in your own life, such as when you're reeling from shocking news or feeling like you can't respond or do anything about a situation.

Thoughts Can Trigger Stress

One of the biggest challenges today is that we constantly face new and unknown threats. Nowadays we rarely come face to face with predators or enemies armed with spears. And being ostracized by a social group doesn't lead to death as it would have for our primitive ancestors. Today's threats often come from within—from our own thoughts. Our brain is not very good at discriminating between actual physical threats and imagined threats. Examples of stressful thoughts could be "What if I'm late for work?" or "I'm not going to make the deadline" or "Dad hasn't called back; what if he's fallen and can't get up?" Compared to physical threats, it's more difficult to tell when the threats that exist only within our minds have been averted. Indeed, can we ever truly get rid of such stressful thoughts? Not even sleep is a safe harbor from negative thoughts. People can live their lives protected from all external physical threats, with a roof over their heads and a rich social life with family and friends, and *still* suffer from anxiety and stress symptoms. Any dog would thrive under the circumstances under which most of us live, but that does not necessarily apply to the human being. Our stress radars are picking up on "threats" from our insides (such as thoughts) or ones that are no longer life threatening (like a deadline at work). How do we deal effectively with such thoughts? This book will help you do just that.

GETTING THINGS DONE: THE ABC LIST AND THE DISTRACTION SHEET

Here we present a method for improving focus and structure when you're about to do something. Part of our memory—the working memory—is highly susceptible to stress (e.g., Arnsten, 2009; Hains et al., 2009) and with all the different channels of information available today, one can easily get distracted and lose focus and feel even more stressed.

The ABC list is a comprehensive to-do list that promotes structure and focus, divided into three parts. *A* stands for the more important tasks, such as a key project, that merit top priority. *B* stands for less important, medium-priority tasks, such as things that should be done within the coming weeks. *C* stands for the least important tasks that are often easy and quick to do but that don't have to get done immediately: answering an email, perhaps, or making a call, looking up something on the Internet, or ordering something. What we tend to do when facing more important tasks or challenges is to spend time on the C tasks, as they don't take much time, energy, and thought. This makes us feel productive, but in a way that overlooks the A and B tasks, which can take longer to do and are more challenging, difficult, and abstract, and thus trigger a stress response. This is where the ABC list can help us see what's most important. Alongside the ABC list, you will use a *distraction sheet*—a blank piece of paper that you keep at your desk (or a blank file on your computer). When you have a thought or an impulse that means having to interrupt your work (to answer an email or do some other nonurgent C task), record it on your distraction sheet instead of following the impulse. Then, when you have a break or have finished what you're doing, you can revisit your distraction sheet and see if you want to add any of these to your ABC list or go ahead and deal with them right away. It's a good idea to use the ABC list daily to prioritize your different tasks. (You can also download the ABC list at the website for this book: http://www.newharbinger.com/41283.)

A The most important tasks, which should be done soon: _____

_____

_____

_____

_____

_____

_____

B The less important tasks, which can be done a bit later: _____

_____

_____

_____

_____

_____

_____

C The least important tasks, which can be done quickly and easily: _____

_____

_____

_____

_____

_____

_____

_____

The Distraction Sheet

When you're trying to focus on an important task and your mind interrupts you and wants you to do something else—look something up on a website, make a phone call, answer a text message (or anything that is not related to the task at hand)—write down the thought and the impulse here. Then continue with your A or B task at hand. When that is done, take a look at your distraction sheet and assign those items to your A, B, or C lists. If they should be done right away, then go ahead with them.

_____

_____

_____

_____

_____

Research in Neuroscience Shows and the Effects of Chronic Stress on the Brain

Using new technology, we can now look inside the brain to gain a better understanding of how it works and discover the links between brain functions, behavior, and mental states.

Chronic stress affects three major regions of the brain (see Figure 2). One is the prefrontal cortex, situated just behind the forehead, which controls decision making, attention regulation, and the inhibition of automatic responses (Arnsten, 2009).

When a person suffers from an acute stress reaction, the prefrontal cortex "goes offline" to some extent, and this negatively affects abstract and flexible thinking. In effect, the brain goes on autopilot. The person does things without thinking and develops tunnel vision.

The second brain region adversely affected by stress is the hippocampus, a seahorse-shaped structure in the middle of the brain, important for learning and in creating memories. Chronic stress and high levels of stress hormones can lead to hippocampal atrophy; the hippocampus may even decrease in size. Loss of memory is therefore common in people who live under stressful conditions for a long time.

The third region of the brain known to be especially sensitive to stress is the amygdala, which plays an important role in processing sensory data and associating them with emotional events—most prominently events triggering fear and terror. While the prefrontal cortex and the hippocampus can deteriorate from prolonged exposure to stress, the amygdala actually becomes more sensitive and more easily triggered, so a person suffering from stress can become prone to fear and anxiety in everyday situations.

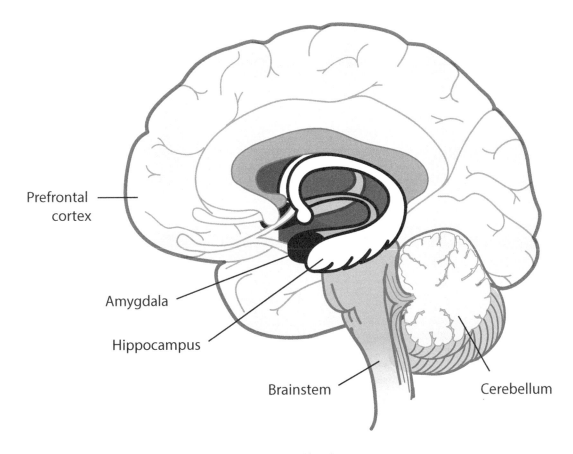

Figure 2: The brain

In this chapter, we noted that humans once needed the physiological energy and psychological focus to handle threats to our very existence. Today, such threats are rare and usually brief. But the brain still has a similar response to stress if we think that something we value (such as our success at work) is threatened. We've discussed the importance of becoming aware of your own stress responses so that you know if they are too overwhelming or go on for too long, so you need to recover.

Over the next week, consider how you recover by taking actions in different areas of your life. What you learn may help you identify those actions that you really enjoy and value. You can then use these actions not only to recover but also to build a life that is more meaningful to you and more balanced. Living a life full of values is very satisfying—and it can help protect you from becoming overwhelmed by the stress you will inevitably experience if you devote too much time and focus on just one of aspect of life that you value. You can then recover from that stress by acting on other values you have previously identified (such as resting and keeping your body healthy).

Congratulations! You've just covered the expanded section of Chapter 1.

CHAPTER 2

What Makes Your Life Meaningful?

The secret to life is meaningless unless you discover it yourself.

—W. Somerset Maugham

At this point you probably have noticed that ACT is very activity based, because it is through the actions you choose to take that you discover what is meaningful to you. You can use these meaningful actions to maintain equilibrium if you tend to focus too exclusively on one value (say, work) or, worse yet, spend time doing activities that give you no value (say, meeting sales targets) or that go against your values (say, stretching the truth to make those targets).

We hope the exercises you worked on over the past week have shown you which activities, in four areas of your life, can help you recharge after stressful times. Now let's review your findings to see if you can identify any actions that may help you recognize your values in each of the four areas. As the Maugham epigraph observes, you can lead a meaningful life only if you discover for yourself what you value, and your actions may help reveal those values to you—or reinforce them.

SO HOW ARE YOU DOING?

Before we proceed with this second chapter's activities, let's follow up on your past week. For each of the following questions, estimate the extent to which you were able to complete each recovery activity, where 0 = not at all and 10 = exactly as planned. Also rate the extent to which you believe each activity helped you to recharge from stress, on a scale from 0 to 10, where 0 = no recharging and 10 = a great deal of recharging.

Activity For each life area, record the recharging activities you undertook since reading Chapter 1	Completed activity: Yes, Partly, or No	Recharging, 0 to 10?

KEY POINTS FROM CHAPTER 1

Different Things Cause Stress

Most people get stressed in new, unpredictable situations in which they feel they have little control, understanding, or ability to manage the situation. Multiple stressful situations in different areas of your life could arise—to give an extreme (but plausible) example, a family member falls ill, you lose your job, and your partner leaves you. These combined circumstances can overwhelm your ability to manage any of them. However, even just one problem in one life area can stress us, particularly when the stressful situation is overwhelming or continues for so long that our body cannot cope with our physiological stress reactions, and we cannot attend to other aspects of life that we value, that give us meaning.

Experiencing Stress Helps with Short-Term Goals, but Harms If We Don't Recharge

When we're faced with multiple, ongoing, pressing demands, there's a strong tendency to devote ourselves more to the imperative ones—those that we *have* to manage (such as taking care of our children). If this devotion mostly prevents us from pursuing other meaningful activities that help us recover and live a more balanced life, then stress and unhappiness may well follow. In the short term, the stress response can be useful by alerting us to a problematic situation, giving us both temporary energy to fulfill an important goal and a fixed focus that allows us solve certain problems. These benefits do not last long, though, as our bodies and minds did not evolve to remain healthy if we do not address a stress response by taking actions that we value in other areas of our life, such as self-care, exercise, and sleep.

CORE SECTION: WHAT MAKES YOUR LIFE MEANINGFUL?

Imagine yourself having a really lousy day. You feel worthless, ugly, washed out, and totally devoid of energy. For once, you have the day off. Now is the perfect time to do something fun, but you're too tired. Just as you've overcome your embarrassment about calling a friend you've been dying to talk to but haven't in ages, you start thinking about the things you *should* be doing instead: clearing out the shed, planning your vacation, finding a plumber. You end up sitting at the kitchen table and staring out the window, frozen in uncertainty about which value is more important at that moment. Oh, and the weather is bleak, and you're wondering why the kitchen doesn't feel as warm lately. After a while, you manage to collect yourself and start sorting the recycling. "Not the best way to spend a day off," you think, "but at least I'm making myself useful."

But are you? Or are you avoiding a difficult activity by doing an easy one, or one that provides you with a quick finish but little life satisfaction? Taking such automatic actions that are not that important at that moment can be a sign of stress: our mind and body losing the ability to act meaningfully. At such times, we may wish to stop ourselves and consider what we'd actually find enjoyable and that could help us recharge our batteries, such as calling family and friends we've been unintentionally ignoring, finding a cat to adopt, or even reading a good novel. In addition, perhaps we have spent so much time on one activity we value (work) that we actually forget we find pleasure in other activities, such as playing card games and doing crossword puzzles. This tends to happen when we overprioritize one, albeit important, life responsibility (such as our small children, sick parents, or work) over other actions (for example, seeing a film, talking with a friend) that can help us recover from overfocusing on only one part of the picture that represents a fulfilling life to us. In short, without taking actions in several dimensions of our lives, we begin to experience a narrow life that constricts us, that we may begin to view as meaningless. At this point we may also experience an existential stress that can turbocharge our stress response. Therefore, it's important to take actions that are important to you in *different areas* of your life, so you can find the joy and vitality you need to focus on tasks that, although meaningful, also tend to cause stress.

We believe that the more activities you try out, the more effective this book will be for you, as one activity we suggest may not resonate with you, but another might. With that in mind, let's try out another activity that highlights the importance of thinking about what is valuable to you and then taking action on it, beginning right now.

Who Are You at Ninety?

Most people know someone who has suffered from a debilitating disease or has been in a serious accident. Faced with the realization that life is fragile and can be shorter than we think, they have changed their life to better align with what is truly important to them. This exercise gives you the chance to get in touch with that sense that life is precarious, to motivate you to consider what really matters to you, without first having to experience a serious accident!

You can listen to a guided version of this exercise on the book's website, http://www.newharbin ger.com/41283, or choose to just read it here. Either way, before beginning, find a place where you can work without any distractions for a few minutes.

All set? Now imagine traveling in time and meeting yourself at the age of ninety, after having lived a life that you have truly valued. Where do you find yourself? Are you in a room or outdoors, in the country or the city, with your grandchildren or with friends? Try to create a picture of your ideal surroundings at that age so you can more easily imagine being there.

Soon you will have visits from three friends or relatives for whom you care deeply. In this future you are imagining, everyone is still alive. This means that even people who've already died, or people who will probably have passed on by the time you reach ninety, can still visit you. These loved ones have come to pay their respects, to tell you what a difference you have made in the lives of those around you, what they feel about you, what you have contributed to them and the world around you. Overall, what do you want them to remember you for? What did you stand for and what values did you follow in life?

For each of the three people, fill in their name and what you would like them to say to you. (Yes, even if you feel you're not currently living up to what you'd like them to say.)

Name: _____

_____

_____

_____

_____

_____

Name: _____

_____

_____

_____

_____

_____

Name: _____

_____

_____

_____

_____

_____

How did it go? Perhaps taking this imaginary trip made you think about those qualities that really matter to *you*, rather than what matters to your visitors. Maybe you haven't thought about these actions and values before. Or maybe you've forgotten about what you valued before you let the stream of life carry you in a direction that, even if considered admirable, you did not mean to prioritize, given how short life is (even if you live to age ninety!).

Thinking about what you really value, while being carried down that stream, can be a bit unpleasant. Maybe you've not found the time (and courage?) to be honest with yourself and to really explore your true values (Dahl, Plumb-Vilardaga, Stewart, & Lundgren, 2009).

You may have realized long ago that striving to live certain values requires that you choose to act in ways that show you prioritize one value over another. These actions may be difficult and stressful; they may take more time than taking the easy way. Are you willing to experience the discomfort and stress that being true to your values may entail? We will show you how you can develop such willingness.

Every action that you take continues to be guided by and reveal what you value. You can never reach your values as an end point, because the picture of your values continues to sharpen and develop until you die. If you value being a loving partner or an outspoken activist, you continue to show those values, perhaps by setting goals that you can accomplish. Those accomplished goals then add up to larger, more complex examples of what you value. When you have (with any luck) reached an advanced age, that direction and those values will be more clear to you as you start painting the picture of who you are, every step of the way.

Your Goals, and How They Relate to Your Values

Values point you to how you might act in every second of your waking life. Wherever you are, you can stop, consider your present situation, and decide to act in accordance with at least one of your values; thus, your behaviors move you in a direction that's true to your values. Alternatively, if you live your life on autopilot, unaware of your current situation, not sure of your values, and guided by avoiding fear, the goals you establish, if any, may paint a blurry picture and your values may seem unclear. So when you set both your short- and long-term goals, choose carefully, bearing in mind what you want your life to be about.

You can also identify subgoals that guide and motivate you to take on more complex actions (say, studying for a degree) that constantly reinforce your progress toward achieving your long-term goals—expanding your knowledge, learning to think critically, and achieving the career that you really want. It has actually been proven that identifying the value of studying for a degree leads to significantly higher grades a year later than just setting goals (Chase et al., 2013).

Now it's time for you to put into practice what we've been saying. What values would you like to emphasize? Which are most important to you? Look at the "homework" you did over the past week, listing the actions that help you recover from life's stresses. Did any of those actions reflect this concept of values? If so, let's emphasize their importance to you by placing them in what we call your Life Compass (see Figure 3). If you like, you can print out blank Life Compass forms—simply visit the book's website, http://www.newharbinger.com/41283, and download the file "LifeCompass.pdf." Or you can just complete the Life Compass form in this book. We'll come back to the Life Compass in all subsequent chapters—it's that important to help you manage stress and live a life of which you are proud—so we recommend that you keep it in a safe place and mark it with pencil, allowing for erasures and updates.

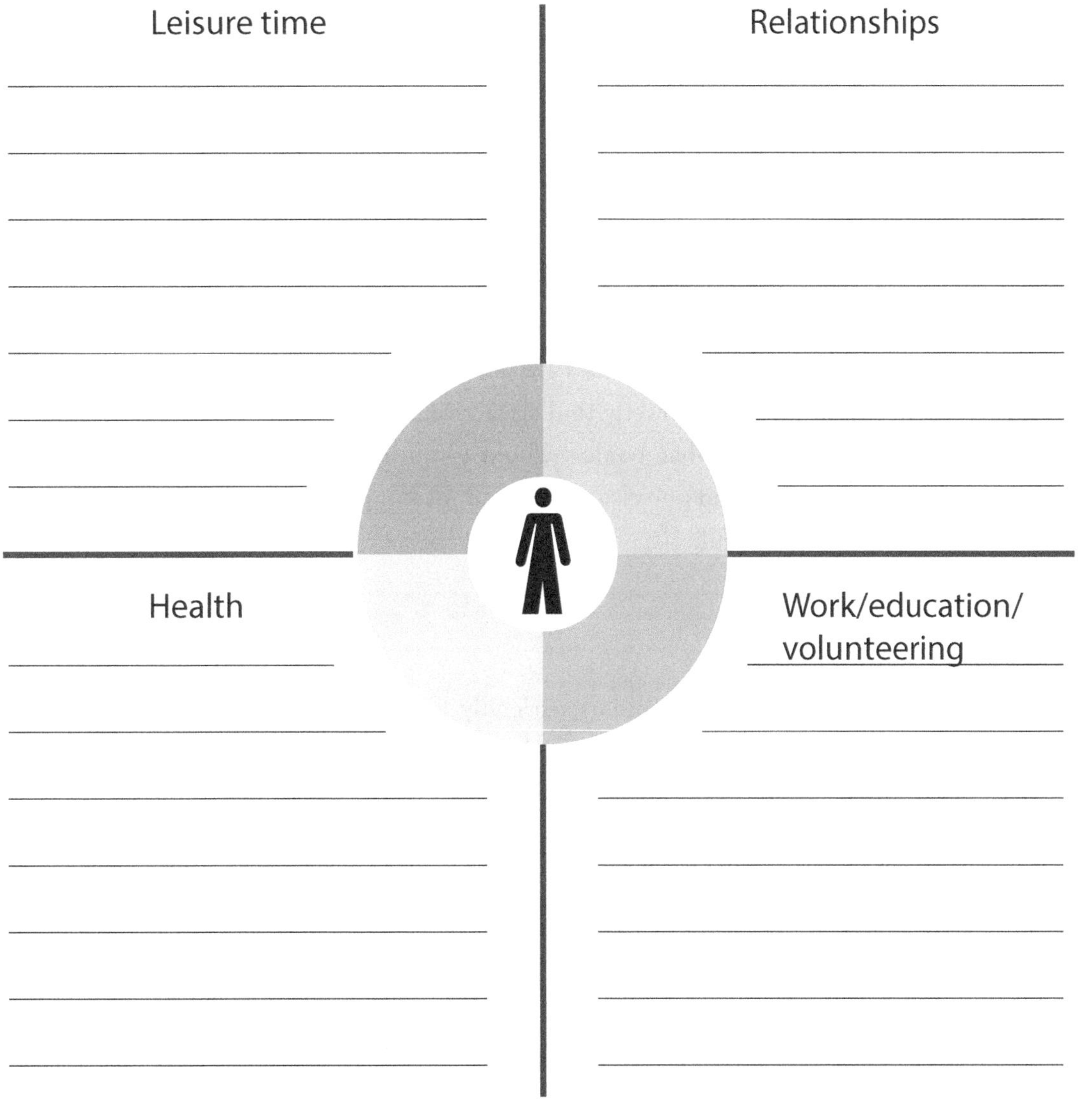

Leisure time

Relationships

Health

Work/education/
volunteering

Figure 3: Life Compass

In the upcoming section "Your Life Compass: Values Examples" we list some aspects or dimensions of life that most people find important. You're welcome to use these as inspirations, and change or tweak them when you fill in your own Life Compass. Please keep in mind that you're the only one who knows what's important to you; thus, to sustain your motivation to let your Life Compass guide you, you should keep it close at hand. These compasses are all too easily set aside, and suddenly you may find yourself going in a direction that is very unappealing to you.

To explore your Life Compass, it can be helpful to imagine that a miracle has occurred, or that you are an all-powerful superhero and anything is possible. What would you do? How would you spend your time? Don't think too hard or overanalyze the possibilities. Just ask yourself what you want your life to be about, and write it down. You can always come back to your notes and revise them later on.

Still unsure how to go about this? No worries—once you've looked at the examples that follow, we're sure you'll get the hang of it pretty quickly.

Your Values Are Your Own

When thinking about what you value, it's important not to think too much about what your culture, society, family, or other people think of you or how they think you "should" or "must" live your life; after all, it's your life, not theirs! Your values are *yours*—not your mom's, your dad's, your political party's, or those of the colleague you secretly find attractive. Simply ask yourself: "If everyone would accept me and love me, no matter what I value, would I still be doing this activity?" This question might help you see what you, and no one else, really find meaningful—what you can pursue to make your life more vital and less stressful.

Your Life Compass

Your Life Compass may look simple and user-friendly, but completing it may be surprisingly challenging. As we've discussed, it asks you to specify the values that will guide your actions. Now, your values and subsequent actions may be similar to those of most people you know. But what if they are not? What if your value of living honestly specifies goals that add up to living openly as transgender? In most societies and cultures, that takes courage to admit. We will teach you skills that can help you cope with the stress that comes with living true to that value. For now, ask yourself what you want from life and what you want to stand for, and write it down on your Life Compass. (We provide some examples that will show you the range of possible values and may start you thinking.) Some actions may reflect several goals, and that's fine; write them down in every relevant part of your life.

Your Life Compass: Values Examples

RELATIONSHIPS

What's important to you when it comes to how, when, and with whom you connect—family, lovers, friends, and the people you see every day (such as while waiting for the 8:25 train)? Forget reality for a minute. Anything is possible! Now, what would you want in your interactions with people? Is there a guiding principle or value for your different behaviors in your different relationships? Kindness, honesty, identifying joint interests? Here are some specific examples; see which resonate with you:

- Being open and vulnerable
- Living a quiet life; not rocking the boat
- Showing appreciation in relationships
- Being able to appreciate the good things in life
- Reaching out to other people
- Being generous
- Taking responsibility, being trustworthy
- Loving and cherishing someone
- Listening without prejudice
- Being open and receptive to people's help and care for me
- Being taken care of
- Letting go
- Respecting others' differences
- Giving someone freedom
- Being honest
- Being courageous
- Letting go of being right

HEALTH

What's important to you when it comes to physical exercise, eating well, and healthy habits? If you could lead the life you dream of, how would you live and act in this area? What would you have to do to cherish your body and spirit? What personal qualities would you need to show?

- Listening to my body

- Giving my body healthy exercise

- Exploring spirituality

- Valuing spending time alone

- Prioritizing myself

- Simple living

- Taking care of my body by eating healthy foods

- Prioritizing a good night's sleep

- Accepting and loving my body despite its limits

- Stopping smoking

- Following a manageable daily routine

- Valuing time off to rest and recharge

LEISURE TIME

What's important to you when it comes to leisure time: hobbies, alone time, spirituality, or community involvement? If you could have everything you had ever dreamed of, how would you live and act in this area? What would you want? What do you like to do in your spare time? Try to describe a perfect afternoon with no work; you can be anywhere you want to be. What's important to you, and what principles would you like to be guided by?

- Personal liberation

- Exploring spirituality

- Being in touch with nature

- Discovering new places

- Finding new ways to relax

- Experiencing a sense of wonder

- Growing as a person

- Challenging myself creatively

- Challenging myself physically

- Seeking adventure

- Enjoying reading

- Prioritizing time with friends

WORK/EDUCATION/VOLUNTEERING

What's important to you when it comes to work, education, self-realization, and developing new skills? If this could include everything you have ever dreamed of for this part of your life, what would you want? Describe a workplace, school, or project with perfect conditions. In an ideal world, how would you like to spend your workday? What's important to you in your work and learning, and what principles would you like to be guided by?

- Evolving

- Learning new things

- Challenging myself

- Working in a balanced way

- Initiating meaningful meetings

- Having fun

- Acting responsibly

- Letting go of obligations

- Working creatively

- Being true to myself

- Taking things lightly

- Being courageous

- Sticking to a schedule

- Practicing acceptance

We hope you are now well on your way in thinking about your own Life Compass. You can come back to the Life Compass as often as you like, to revise or add to it.

Helpful Tips and Frequently Asked Questions for Filling Out the Life Compass

Should I just write down the things I value in my life right now, or should I also include things I want to work for in the future?

Write down everything you feel is important in the life you are living now and the things you want to bring into your life. Also, some things may already be locked into place; others aren't quite there yet, although you'd love to make them a bigger part of your life. Don't feel limited by your present: in an ideal world, what would you like to fill your life with?

I don't know what I want! Please, help me!

It's not always easy to differentiate between what *you* want and what *others* want from you. Worse yet, we may take on other people's values for fear of not being accepted and fitting in. Ironically, acting in such ways often leads to a life worthy of a starring role in English Victorian literature, in which you, as the main character, live for others, ignore your own desires, and die sad and alone. Is this what you want for your life? If not, be brave. Try out the things you've always wanted to, but haven't. Do this often and, without overthinking it, see what brings the most meaning for you in your life. It's a process of trial and error that may always be a work in progress. Just keep trying until you find actions that are meaningful to you.

Filling out the Life Compass makes me sad. Why is that?

It's not unusual to feel blue or even sad when filling out the Life Compass. There are a number of reasons for this. A common one is seeing a discrepancy between your ideal life and the life you're actually leading. In this case, any confusion, anxiety, pain, or grief are your friends. They can motivate you to make changes to your life!

I'm not sure if all fields in the Life Compass are relevant to me. Is that normal?

The four Life Areas in the Life Compass are generally seen as important to most people, but the emphasis placed on each individual area varies from person to person and over the course of each life. Remember, there is no right or wrong here. If you're a parent, for example, it is not uncommon to put extra emphasis on relationships, and perhaps deemphasize work as you once knew it (that is, in an office, outside of the home). Once the kids are in school or grown up, you may find work becoming more important to you.

Deathbed Regrets

Another way of looking at values is identifying regrets for what you did or didn't do. In the book *The Top Five Regrets of the Dying*, author and nurse Bronnie Ware lets us know the most common regrets of people on their deathbed. Over many years of providing palliative care, she was able to identify several common themes. We list the most common themes she recorded. Read through and see if any of these resonate with you. If so, how might they inform goals that help you move your life toward your values?

I wish I'd had the courage to live a life true to myself, not the life others expected of me. When people realized that their life was almost over and reflected on it, it was easy for them to see how many dreams had gone unfulfilled. They found they had lived a life based on other people's expectations and had not followed most of their own dreams.

I wish I hadn't worked so hard. Many patients had worked hard and regretted missing out on their children's youth and having a more intimate relationship with their partner.

I wish I'd had the courage to express my feelings. Many had suppressed their true feelings to keep peace with others. Or they'd neglected to tell other people how much they loved and cared for them. These patients had settled for a mediocre existence and never explored the full potential of a number of relationships. Men, in particular, are often fearful of expressing or even allowing themselves to feel their emotions.

I wish I had stayed in touch with my friends. Many people had become so caught up in their own lives that they had let friendships deteriorate over the years. There were many regrets about not giving friendships the time and effort that they deserved. Some friends had already passed away, and others were difficult to find.

I wish that I had let myself be happier. Many did not realize until the end that, to some extent, happiness is a choice that often comes from seeing how you can take meaningful action, even when you feel low. They got stuck in old behavior patterns and habits. The smothering, constricting comfort of familiarity was allowed to rule their lives, and they regretted not breaking out of their comfort zone.

Do these deathbed regrets resonate with you at all? Are they helpful in identifying the things that matter to you? Did you find anything to add to your Life Compass? If so, add your findings to your Life Compass or write them down here:

Relationships: _____

_____

Leisure time: _____

_____

Health: _____

_____

Work/education/volunteering: _____

_____

NOW THAT YOU KNOW YOUR VALUES

Once you have defined what matters most to you, you can start taking small steps toward living a life more in tune with your own wishes. Look around and see what actions you can take now that represent your values. Only by changing your everyday behavior can you live the life that you want. In the pages to come, we will give you tips on how to establish concrete goals that allow you to live the values that may give your life meaning and satisfaction. Start by taking a look at Angela's list of values and the concrete behaviors that reflect those values. Like Angela, you can try to identify small steps in your daily life that are connected to your values and write them down in the empty spaces of the Concrete Behaviors Compass that follows.

Example: Angela's Values and Concrete Behaviors

Value	Concrete Behavior
Personal liberation	Take a walk during my lunch break, even if thoughts of work still pop into my head.
	Try walking a new route each week and exploring new places.
Listening to my body	Sit down for a minute when I get home.
	Take short breaks.
	Eat healthier food in smaller portions.
Standing up for myself at work	Don't automatically accept new assignments; ask for time to think about how they might help me in my career plan.
	Use my personal time at work for a workout.
Being open and vulnerable	Tell my husband that I love him.
	Tell my friend what she means to me.
Letting go of obligations	Split kitchen duties 50/50 with my husband.
	Tell colleagues to ask for help when they need it. I need to give up trying to control everyone.

Your Concrete Behaviors

Fill in the blank Concrete Behaviors Compass (see Figure 4) with small actions you can take that represent each of the four dimensions of your life. Take your time—don't rush this. Keep in mind, you're defining concrete actions that can provide long-term, or even immediate, benefits to your life. If you like, you can print out blank compass forms; simply visit the book's website, http://www.newharbinger.com/41283, to download the file. Post them where you can see them, fold them up and put them in your wallet, or keep them in your smartphone so they're always close at hand, to remind you how you could act at any moment to give meaning to your life. For additional tips, read the expanded section of this chapter or take a look at Angela's compasses at the end of the core section that follows.

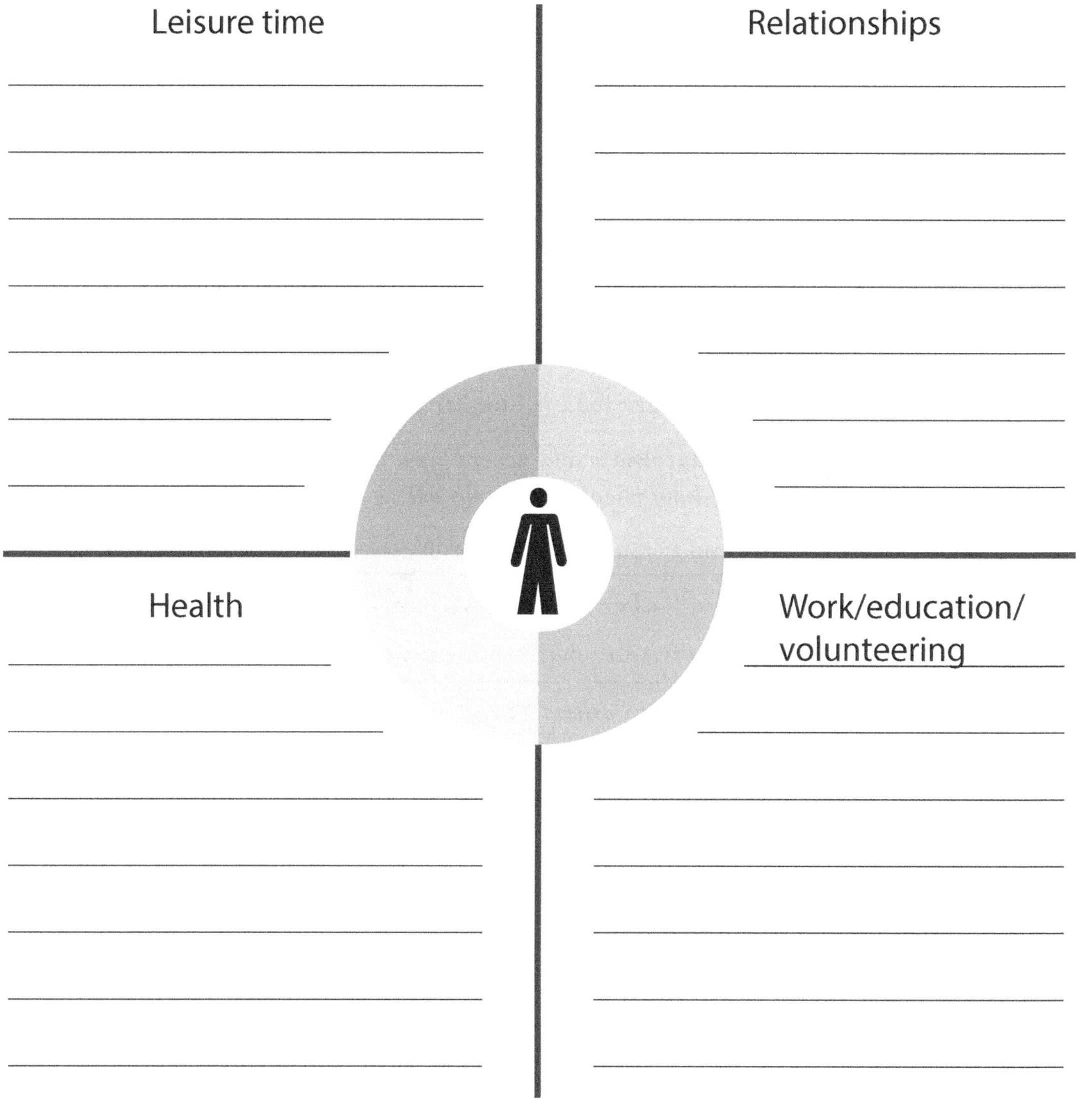

Leisure time

Relationships

Health

Work/education/
volunteering

Figure 4: Concrete Behaviors Compass

Picking a Value and Taking Concrete Steps

Now pick a value and one or two concrete behaviors that you associate with that value—preferably something you have time to do this week or before you read the next chapter. Write down your choices and schedule the activity or behavior on your calendar. Set an alarm on your smartphone or write yourself a note and post it where you can see it.

Value to focus on before reading the next chapter: _____

Concrete steps: _____

_____

_____

_____

TAKING ACTION: WHAT YOU CAN DO BEFORE READING THE NEXT CHAPTER

Here are some activities we suggest you do before moving on to the next chapter. Your values are revealed in your actions, so we would like you to:

Embrace a value. Make time for taking at least one concrete action toward a life value; any action toward an appropriate value you've listed will do. You shouldn't expect to run before you can walk, so you may wish to build your confidence by choosing a concrete action that will not cause you too much stress or take more time than you reasonably have.

Recharge. Schedule and carry out at least one recharging activity.

Read on. Schedule a day for reading Chapter 3 of this book. About a week from now would be ideal. Make a note in your calendar or set an alarm on your phone.

FOLLOW JOHN AND ANGELA IN THEIR EFFORTS TO LIVE A MORE MEANINGFUL AND BALANCED LIFE

Angela's Life Compass

Leisure time

Personal liberation.

Appreciating the beautiful things in life.

Enjoying the smaller things.

Relationships

Being open and vulnerable.

Letting go of obligations.

Being honest.

Accepting help from others.

Health

Listening to my body.

Healthy eating.

Working out.

Work/education/ volunteering

Standing up for myself at work.

Learning new things.

Solving problems at work.

Finding balance at work.

Angela's To-Do List Before Reading the Next Chapter

Value to embrace before reading the next chapter: *Finding balance at work.*

Concrete steps: *Find someone to help out with pastries on Fridays or stop baking altogether.*

Angela's Life Compass

Leisure time

Book a trip with a friend every six months.

Remind myself to enjoy my cup of coffee.

Take in the scenery during walks.

Listen to my old records.

Relationships

Reconnect with Beth and other friends to

tell them I miss them.

Schedule a girls' night out.

Ask Alicia if she wants to take evening

walks with me.

Health

Go swimming once a week.

Eat slowly, with screens turned off.

Go to bed at the same time each night.

Set the alarm on weekends instead

of sleeping in.

Work/education/ volunteering

Prioritize my work goals with my boss,

Use my break time at work for a workout;

ask Anne to come along.

Find a training course I want to take;

show my boss.

Find someone to help out with pastries

on Fridays, or stop baking altogether.

All of us are programmed (unknowingly) with rules: instructions by which to live, such as "You must always do your best." These rules are simple and direct; they say we *must* do something or we *have to* do something. These strict rules sometimes help us live a vital life, but they often become obstacles. Read the expanded section to find out more about these rules and how you can prevent them from living the life you want to live! Since stress and insomnia are closely related, we will also provide you with tools for better sleep in the expanded section.

CHAPTER 2 EXPANDED SECTION

Our well-learned rules can prevent us from living our values and can promote stress. (Perhaps we should consider retiring them?)

All that has happened in your life you carry with you—as memories, as inclinations to act in certain ways, and as views of the world and yourself. You can call it your backpack of experiences. What you learn from the things you have experienced forms a code you could call "rules" or "life rules." They are the ways you look at the world and yourself; they affect how you behave and what you do. Rules are the product of your history; they represent what your parents, teachers, and society have taught you. In many ways, they form an important part of you. But will the "you" that has formed help you to live as the "you" that you wish to be? Will the rules, thoughts, and emotions that your past has given you help you live meaningfully now and in the future? Sometimes the rules that you rigidly follow prevent you from living your values; instead, they promote stress. Examples of these rigid rules could be "I have to be perfect in whatever I do"; "No one is ever here to help me, I have to take care of myself"; "I'm the one who must take responsibility for this; otherwise, nothing will happen"; and "No matter how busy I am, I must always make time for others."

When your personal rules contain words such as "should," "have to," and "must," they seem like a universal law of the universe (Newton would probably not agree they are!) that you are obligated to follow. But however ingrained these early learned rules are, with practice you can recognize them and then choose whether to follow them or not, based on the control you now have over your actions.

If you feel that your life is filled to the brim with obligations, musts, and have-to's, you need to stop for a minute and think about what you could let go of. Or could these obligations actually be connected to your values, the things that matter to you? Let's have a look at your musts and have-to's.

EXERCISE: STRESSFUL RULES AND OBLIGATIONS

What rigid rules or obligations are you using to trip yourself up on? Try to think of a few situations where you usually tell yourself that you are obligated to do something, and write them in the table. By answering the following questions you can figure out whether they are values you want to follow or rigid rules you have learned. Sometimes you can spot one of these rules when you fear that "if I don't do X, then Y (something bad) will happen."

Take a look at Angela's completed example:

Rules or obligations I follow that cause stress	*"I have to take time to listen to my colleagues at work, even though I am busy."*
Is this a law of the universe or is it actually something you choose to do?	*Well, It's a choice! Even though it feels like it's a must or almost a law of nature.*
Why do you do it? (To avoid some potential negative outcome? Because you're following a value of yours? Or both?)	Avoiding negative outcomes *I'm afraid people will not talk to me if I am not super friendly and attentive.* Value *It's also a value; I value connecting to people.*
What value of yours could guide you in approaching this situation differently to lower stress?	Values *Taking care of myself.* *Connecting to people.*
How could you approach this situation in a new way to lower stress?	*I can tell my self that I **choose** to connect; it's not a must!* *I can connect to people **when I want to** and have time, not as an automatic thing I **have** to do.*

On the next page is a blank table for you to fill in.

Rules or obligations I follow that cause stress	
Is this a law of the universe or is it actually something you choose to do?	
Why do you do it? (To avoid some potential negative outcome? Because you're following a value of yours? Or both?)	Avoiding negative outcomes Value
What value of yours could guide you in approaching this situation differently to lower stress?	Values
How could you approach this situation in a new way to lower stress?	

The next time you feel the weight of an obligation, try to figure out why you've chosen to meet it. See if you can identify an underlying value that leads you to *choose* to meet it and approach it in a way that gives you more wiggle room.

Tools for Better Sleep

Stress and insomnia are closely related. Too little sleep makes us more susceptible to stress; it dampens our spirit and eventually makes us more likely to become depressed, anxious, or angry. Recent findings have shown several benefits of giving sleep a high priority and giving ourselves the nightly rest we need. For most people, this means seven to eight hours of sleep a night (Åkerstedt, Kecklund, Alfredsson, & Selen, 2007; Van Cauter & Spiegel, 1999; Morin et al., 2006).

If you have serious difficulty sleeping, you should contact a doctor and consider finding a CBT course or self-help book that directly target sleep problems, such as *The Sleep Book: How to Sleep Well Every Night* (2014) by sleep expert Dr. Guy Meadows. However, the following advice and tips can be a good start. We also present a sleep journal shortly, which can be helpful.

The following tips have been shown to be helpful for a good night's sleep—if you follow them. (The tips are numbered for reference later; their order is not important.) Circle the areas that are especially appropriate for you and that you would like to try out.

1. *Go to bed at the same time every night.* Going to bed and getting up at roughly the same times every day can prove beneficial. One way to find out how much you actually sleep (as opposed to how much you *think* you sleep) is to use the sleep journal or one of the many apps available.

2. *Make time for sleep.* In other words, make sure you set aside enough hours for sleeping. Don't let anything else get in the way.

3. *Wind down.* We can easily find ourselves working or doing other pulse-raising activity right up until we go to bed. When we do, the brain is still fully activated and we find it hard to settle. Spend at least one and a half hours before bedtime doing something relaxing and calming.

4. *Keep your bedroom a bedroom.* We can easily work and do other "wakeful" activities in bed, which means that in the end we stop associating the bed with rest and sleep. Sex, reading, and other calming activities will promote sleep—plowing through your inbox probably won't. Clear the bedroom of everything that isn't conducive to sleep.

5. *Avoid evening stimulants.* Coffee, tea, cocoa, alcohol, and nicotine affect our activation system in different ways. Caffeine takes a long time to leave the body, so it's best to avoid tea and coffee for five hours before bed. Don't drink alcohol in the last few hours either— even though it can make it easier to drop off, it interferes with the quality of your sleep.

6. *Be physically active.* Do your best to get regular exercise. Apart from generally lowering our stress levels and burning energy (not to mention the health benefits), it also makes us better at regulating our body temperature, which is good for sleep.

7. *Use daylight.* Try to get some daylight. It "sets" our biological clock and helps regulate the body's circadian rhythm. When you must be indoors, try to sit by the window in your office, classroom, or wherever else you sit during the day.

8. *Avoid sleeping during the day.* If you sleep during the day you may find it harder to drop off at night. If you're really tired, try a relaxation exercise or take a short nap of no longer than twenty minutes. If you do sleep well at night and have the opportunity to take daytime naps, that can be a healthy habit.

9. *Keep a notebook by your bed.* Niggling thoughts are a common cause of insomnia. Some people find it helpful to write down their worries or ideas so they can be retrieved later.

10. Try not to worry about not sleeping. Anxiety about not being able to sleep can keep us awake! Remember, though, that the brain and body are perfectly able to cope with a temporary lack of sleep, which the brain compensates for with more deep sleep. Even though most of us benefit from seven to eight hours of sleep a night, needs vary, and we're all different. Don't feel that you have to live up to some imaginary norm about what constitutes a good night's sleep.

11. *Establish an evening ritual.* The body and its circadian rhythm benefit from routines. When we follow a certain routine before we go to bed, we send a signal to the body that it's soon time to sleep.

12. *Avoid heavy meals before bedtime.* A large evening meal activates the digestive system and makes it harder for you to fall asleep; it can also affect the quality of sleep you eventually get.

13. *Don't go to bed hungry.* Your hungry body will have trouble relaxing, as it's hardwired to satisfy that craving. A light snack of easily digestible food an hour before bedtime is ideal.

14. *If you wake up in the night, don't eat, and drink only water.* Eating or drinking anything with calories can activate your body and disrupt your sleep rhythm. If you're thirsty, it's okay to drink water. But if you've been awakened by hunger pangs and really need to quell them, as with late-evening snacks, make it light and easily digestible.

15. *Use a good alarm clock.* To eliminate any anxiety about not waking up on time, use a reliable alarm clock (and even set a backup if it makes you feel more comfortable).

In addition to these tips, you might want to try our sleep journal. You can also visit http://www.newharbinger.com/41283 to download the journal, along with a useful plan.

Even if you don't have trouble sleeping but would like to test some of our advice, you can jot down the ones you'd like to try here. It's also a good idea to enter a reminder in your calendar or phone.

_____

_____

_____

_____

How to Use a Sleep Journal

Insomnia has a wide variety of causes and often accompanies other problems. When we're having difficulties and our sleep is affected, we can end up in a vicious cycle of mutually reinforcing states. When we make sure that we have time to get a good night's sleep, we benefit in other ways too.

Completing a sleep journal will make it easier for you to monitor whether your sleep is affected by the advice you follow. We suggest that you write in your journal as soon as you wake up in the morning. If you've had periods of sleep and wakefulness, it can be hard to estimate times, but do your best—this isn't an exact science. Skip any lines that aren't relevant.

Change takes time; if our advice doesn't work for you right away, don't give up. After a few weeks, refer to your sleep journal to see how you're doing.

Sleep Journal

	Monday	Tuesday	Wednesday	Thursday	Friday	Saturday	Sunday
Went to bed at ____ o'clock:							
Fell asleep after roughly ____ minutes:							
Woke up ____ times and stayed awake for ____ minutes:							
Woke up at ____ o'clock:							
Got up at ____ o'clock:							
Yesterday, slept ____ minutes/hours during the day:							
Total of ____ hours' sleep last night:							
How well did I sleep last night?*							
Sleeping tips I used (1–15)							

* 1 = terribly, 2 = quite badly, 3 = neither badly nor well, 4 = quite well, 5 = like a baby

In this chapter's core section, you began gaining some clarity on your values and what could make your life more true to them and more meaningful. If you also read the expanded section, you took a look at "life rules" you may have been following and considered whether they have held you back from your potential life of meaning, and you added some tools for better sleep.

In the next chapter, we'll explore mindfulness—a technique that can help you rid yourself of the armor that prevents you from acting now to create the tomorrow that you value. In the chapters to come you will begin to use mindfulness, willingness, and compassion to experience each present moment and the different internal responses that accompany them. As you do, we invite you to be open, without judgment, to all the feelings that come and go with each passing moment—even the fears and suffering, the frustrations and regrets. By embracing with compassion the "I" that your history has fashioned, you can free yourself from simply enduring or avoiding much of the stress associated with your past. And you can take actions today to create the willingness and courage to boldly take the path of a meaningful life, regardless of the challenges that await you on that journey.

Mindfulness: Creating Meaning and Reducing Stress in the Present and Future

Mindfulness is simply being aware of what is happening right now without wishing it were different; enjoying the pleasant without holding on when it changes (which it will); being with the unpleasant without fearing it will always be this way (which it won't).

—James Baraz

As we noted at the end of the last chapter, mindfulness can help us identify, prioritize, and find the energy and courage to pursue our values. In addition, mindfulness itself can reduce stress (O'Leary, O'Neill, & Dockray, 2015; Chiesa & Serretti, 2009), but we want to encourage you to use it primarily to enhance your willingness to experience the difficult feelings that will inevitably arise when you pursue a meaningful life. Thinking of mindfulness this way will help you live a vital life, *and* this life will not be as stressful—vital, and certainly challenging, but not crushing and forever exhausting. So let's make a start!

SO HOW ARE YOU DOING?

Before we proceed with this third chapter's activities, let's follow up on your past week. For each of the following two questions, estimate the extent to which you were able to complete the activity, where Yes = exactly as planned and No = not at all. Also rate the extent to which you believe each activity helped you recover from stress, on a scale from 0 to 10, where 0 = no recovery and 10 = a great deal of recovery.

Activity	Completed?			Recovery, 0 to 10?
Took a small step on the basis of a value	Yes	Partly	No	
Did at least one recovery activity	Yes	Partly	No	

Mindfulness is an essential tool that can lead us to live a life that we value. To what extent have you been leading such a life? Let's use the Life Compass to help answer that question.

On the Life Compass, the 0 to 10 scale along each arrow relates to how many actual steps you've taken in this area over the past week: the more steps, the higher the score. The scale is completely subjective; it is about how *you* want to live your life, not what other people think or tell you how you *ought* to live it. If you're a single parent with two children and a full-time job, maybe you'll give yourself a score of 10 under "Relationships" for having called two friends during the week. If you're single without children, maybe a score of 10 represents having met up with three friends. You decide what's appropriate for your circumstances.

Give yourself a mark for your score in each area, factoring in everything you identified as important earlier. Think also in terms of quality and quantity. For example, say that a value for you is "taking care of my body," and one concrete step in this direction is to go to the gym. Say that you've gone to the gym every day this week, but that you've done so beating yourself up that you're an ugly pig. As you work out, you've been hard on yourself and stressed your way through the session instead of being present to it. In this case, the quantity was high but the quality low, so an honest overall score might be low.

After rating yourself in each area, you can connect all your scores with a loop. It could look something like the example here.

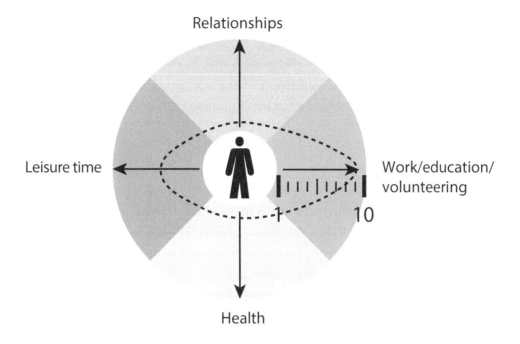

What does your Life Compass look like the past week? Fill in this blank compass.

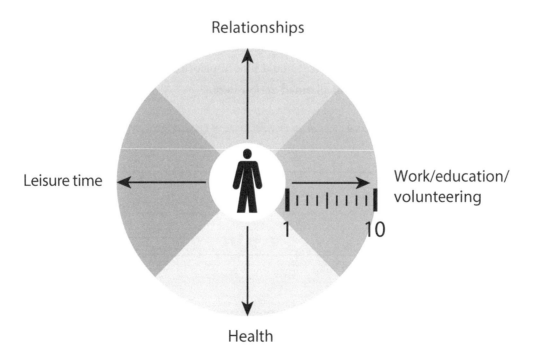

Well done! Your compass gives you the following two important pieces of information:

Life Space

Imagine that you're standing in the middle of the compass. If there's a lot of space between you and the loop you've drawn, you've been acting in ways that you value—meaning you've given yourself a generous life space that allows you to thrive! If there is little space around you, you might not be taking the necessary actions that allow you to live a meaningful life true to your values and thereby alleviate stress.

Balance

If the loop you've drawn is circular, essentially like a wheel, your life will roll along more smoothly down the path of meaning and vitality that you've chosen. If it's uneven, don't worry, it's perfectly normal. Different life demands require our attention from week to week. But if the imbalance persists, it might feel as if you have acted meaningfully in one area at the cost of ignoring other values you have. You begin feeling stressed, and maybe devoid of meaning, and maybe ashamed of yourself for ignoring relationships you value. This stress is not easy to acknowledge, so you may ignore the signs of it that we discussed earlier, until your body fails you, or other meaningful aspects of your life are about to die on the vine. Maybe it's time to change something? Ironically, the solution to imbalance is usually to do *more*—that is, more of whatever provides you with recovery; more of something you're not currently doing; more that will make your Life Compass rounder. This, of course, includes taking breaks, resting, sleeping, and so on.

Going by what your Life Compass currently looks like, is there anything you'd want to do more or less of over the coming week? Some area you'd like to prioritize? It's best to take a small step, not an overly challenging one. Write your planned action here.

_____

_____

_____

_____

KEY POINTS FROM CHAPTER 2

Not Following Your Life's Values Can Cause Stress

When we're stressed, we tend to do more of the "shoulds" and "musts" and cut down on the things that allow us to recover and all the other things that give meaning to our lives. Losing our compass direction like this not only prevents recovery but also can lead to an unfulfilled life or a life devoid of meaning. You can call it "existential stress."

The Life Compass Can Help Us Get Back on Track

With a simple Life Compass we can give ourselves time to think about the most important things in our lives. Our greatest chance of success in achieving a meaningful life is to focus on our own actions and what we can do to align our life more according to our Life Compass.

Values Are Not Goals

"Values" is the term we use to refer to what's most important in our lives. Values differ from goals in that they're never attained once and for all. Goals, like "buying a house," can be ticked off a list, but a value like "creating a sense of security" can guide our actions over and over again in daily life. Goals are in the future (until we reach them); values are always in the present.

CORE SECTION: STARTING WHERE YOU ARE, HERE AND NOW

As we mentioned in Chapter 2, short-term stress is a part of living a vital, fulfilling life. If the stress goes on too long, though, our bodies may not physically cope well, and we experience unwanted emotions, because we are not taking sufficient action to experience value in other areas of our life; this in turn further exacerbates our stress. So we need to take action to let our body recover in the service of being healthy, and we may need to also do something in another area of our life to achieve a greater diversity of meaning, which will not only bring us satisfaction but also help inoculate us against future stress. We may need to occasionally take a good look at our lives and start prioritizing values that we then commit to pursuing. This may mean, for example, that at times we work a bit less so we can sustain and build our relationships and health.

Mindfulness: Being Present to the Here and Now

Although almost all of the major religions use practices that we can interpret as facilitating mindfulness, we do not link mindfulness to any religion. We use mindfulness as an evidence-based technique, a useful way of approaching life that any person can understand and benefit from, whatever the person's religious or nonreligious background or present circumstances. Mindfulness is an active attitude and a technique for letting your thoughts be and returning to what you are experiencing in the here and now—not pushing anything away, nor pulling anything toward you; just being here with an open, nonjudgmental attitude. There are many definitions of mindfulness and just as many ways to practice it. We like this definition by Kabat-Zinn (2005): "Mindfulness can be thought of as moment-to-moment, nonjudgmental awareness, cultivated by paying attention in a specific way, that is, in the present moment, and as nonreactively, as nonjudgmentally, and as openheartedly as possible."

A great way to learn is by doing, so let us begin to experience mindfulness in this chapter's exercises.

MINDFULNESS CAN HELP US SEE THOUGHTS AS THOUGHTS

One way to begin practicing mindfulness is to realize that you are actually thinking! Your thoughts can get in the way of living a life that you value. One of the brain's tasks is to produce thoughts, and research shows (and you can likely affirm) that many of these are negative. If the thought "I'm a fraud" comes into your mind, you might experience it without questioning it; you respond to it as a reality, which is not useful to you, because your thoughts can influence your behavior. If you accept the thought as truth, it will probably affect things you do. You might try to pretend to be "good," to boast and exaggerate. Or you might avoid doing things so as not to be "exposed" as the imposter you think you are. If, on the other hand, you maintain a mindful and healthy distance from your thoughts, you are more free to act as you wish. You are viewing the thought for the thought it is. Maybe distressing, maybe interesting, but nonetheless just a thought. Yes, thoughts can stress you, and as we've said, the brain is not that good at telling an imaginary threat from a real one.

EXERCISE: I'M HAVING THE THOUGHT THAT …

This exercise is a simple way of creating a healthy distance from your thoughts. When you become aware of what you're thinking, you can precede the thought with the phrase "I'm having the thought that …"

Try this and see if you notice any difference. First read the following sentence carefully and think about it:

"I'm a failure."

Then read this sentence carefully and think about it:

"I'm having the thought that I'm a failure."

No doubt you found it easier to see the second sentence as a thought, and a less potent one. When you tell yourself things like "I'm a failure," you make a value judgment. Even if it might feel true, or you could find "proof" for it by comparing yourself with others, your being a "failure" is not a fact. "Failure" is not an inherent characteristic, merely a judgment statement produced by using language.

To reduce your thoughts' power over you, try this next exercise.

First, decide how much time you want to devote to it. Let's say three minutes. Note in the following spaces as many thoughts as you can during this time. You might write something about:

- The thoughts passing through your head.

- Difficult thoughts that you might not be having right now but that your brain can sometimes produce.

- Nice thoughts that you might not be having right now but that your brain can sometimes produce. (Judgmental thoughts can be both negative and positive.)

Don't worry about how "true" these thoughts are; just jot them down as thoughts.

Start your timer, and off you go!

I'm having the thought that _____

_____

_____

I'm having the thought that _____

_____

_____

I'm having the thought that _____

_____

_____

I'm having the thought that _____

_____

_____

I'm having the thought that _____

_____

_____

I'm having the thought that _____

_____

_____

Time's up! How did you experience this exercise? In relationship to your thoughts, was there any difference, even slight, from how you normally see them?

_____

_____

If you didn't feel a bit more distance between you and your thoughts, don't worry. This recording exercise takes time to practice, and we have more exercises ahead to guide you through. We have recorded specific audio exercises that are a part of this program (available at http://www.newharbinger.com/41283), and before the next chapter you will have more chances to practice and understand mindfulness.

We suggest you keep this phrase with you as a companion in everyday life: "I am having the thought that …" This can help you build your skills of *seeing* your thoughts rather than *being* your thoughts.

Now it's time for another mindfulness exercise: "Three Things."

EXERCISE: THREE THINGS

It's effective to practice mindfulness one sense at a time. The human body has five physical senses: taste, hearing, touch, vision, and smell (acknowledging those who are differently abled). Apart from perceiving our world through whichever of these senses we have, we also experience feelings and thoughts.

When we practice mindfulness in our daily lives, we can enlist the help of our physical senses by being mindful of them one at a time. Let us show you what we mean with the "Three Things" exercise. (You'll also find this exercise recorded at http://www.newharbinger.com/41283.)

1. Make sure you can sit undisturbed for three minutes.

2. Settle down in a chair.

3. Start by taking note of three different things you can see. Really look at them, one at a time.

4. Now shut your eyes and take note of three different sensations in your body—perhaps what you can feel at three different areas of your body—again, one at a time. Stay open, inviting any sensation, even if it is uncomfortable.

5. Now take note of three different sounds you can hear—again, one at a time, without judging.

6. Repeat steps 3 through 5, but this time take note of just *two* things you can see, feel, and hear.

7. Now repeat steps 3 through 5, but each time with only one thing.

This exercise is easy to do during a break at work or when you're sitting on the bus or the train. It develops your ability to focus and be present in the here and now with an open attitude.

MINDFULNESS ON THE GO!

You can tap into mindfulness at most points during your busy day, both to reduce stress and to identify and prioritize your values-based activities. Many people find the following mindfulness exercises useful.

EXERCISE: LISTEN MINDFULLY TO MUSIC

This different way of listening to music can help you be nonjudgmentally mindful of what you're listening to.

1. Choose a piece of music at random. It could be familiar music, or music that you never normally listen to, or a piece that you've never heard before.

2. Turn on your stereo or put your headset on and allow yourself to be consumed by the instruments, the voices (if any), and the tunes. Pay attention to the details instead of the whole composition; notice the beat, the rhythm, the light or dark tones, the salient instruments, the loudest background instruments, whatever. Try attending to one thing at a time; for example, you could concentrate on one instrument for a while, then switch to another.

3. If judgmental thoughts and feelings emerge, such as "This is awful" or "This isn't my kind of music," simply take note of these thoughts and feelings and open yourself fully to the music again. Allow yourself to become fully immersed in every detail of the music.

We each learn things differently; some people master a skill by doing something one way, while others use a different technique. Thus, the more mindfulness techniques you try, the better the chance you will find one, or a combination, that works for you. So let's try another one.

EXERCISE: BRINGING MINDFUL ATTENTION TO WHATEVER YOU ARE UP TO

At any time of day you can practice bringing your attention to what you are doing and focus your attention on any one of the five senses. When walking, you can feel your feet or legs moving; when showering, you can feel the water against your skin; when brushing your teeth, you can feel the brush in your hand and mouth. When you're in a more active situation, such as with a child, you might have to make a particular effort to just be "extra present." At such times it can be difficult to focus on one sense at a time, but it is possible to be present to touch, vision, thoughts, and feelings. You can remind yourself to return to the present moment when your thoughts start to drift away to something else. Here are some examples of candidates—everyday activities it's likely you do relatively regularly in a normal week.

Eating breakfast	Exercising	Having a conversation
Doing the dishes	Walking upstairs	Brushing teeth
Showering	Getting dressed	Walking
Driving	Waking up	Riding on a bus, train, bike
Watching something	Eating dinner	Drinking
Washing hands	Going to bed	Being with children

Other:

Circle one or more of these activities if you'd like to try practicing mindfulness this way the coming week, or choose your own activity. When you practice mindfulness during one of these activities, here are some things you might find helpful:

1. Write down the activity you've chosen for this week in a place you'll see it: your calendar or the kitchen table. Try sticking a little colored note in the place where you normally do the activity.

2. During your activity, let your mind be present in one or several of the five senses, and let yourself experience the moment in each one of them, one at a time. Do your best to stay open, inviting even the uncomfortable sensations, without judging them.

3. Take note of what you experience in that present moment, gently bringing your attention back to the present moment when inevitably it drifts.

Tip: Perhaps saying to yourself "I, here, now …" will help bring you into the present moment.

Example: In the Shower

I, here, now … can feel the shower floor tiles under my feet.

I, here , how … can feel the warm water on my skin.

I, here, now … am reaching for the shampoo.

When your thoughts start to wander, become aware of this and allow yourself to return gently to the present:

"I, here, now … realize that I'm planning tonight's dinner, and I'm going to choose to bring my attention back to taking my shower."

And now to another practical skill: mindful breathing

YOU CAN ALWAYS BREATHE MINDFULLY (YOU WON'T DISTURB ANYONE)

As you know, in stressful situations your breathing can often become fast and shallow, and this type of breathing can become the norm for people who experience chronic stress. This shallow breathing in turn leads to even more stress, strain, and muscle tension. When you breathe mindfully, you tend to have a more harmonious and rhythmic breathing pattern that can increase your chances of recovery, relieve muscle tension, and bring a full supply of oxygen to your bloodstream. A deep breath should be long and slow, activating your abdomen and your chest all the way up to your collarbone.

Let's try to move from this shallow breathing to a more useful, mindful breathing pattern. The following two exercises can help you do that.

EXERCISE: SLOW FULL BREATHING

We recommend starting with a simple exercise that takes less than sixty seconds. You can do it any time, any place. (This exercise is also available at http://www.newharbinger.com/41283.)

1. Let your attention go to your abdomen; just feel your abdomen.
2. Relax your abdomen, letting it be soft; no tightening or holding in.
3. Slowly inhale a deep breath through your nostrils, filling your lungs from the bottom up: first let your abdomen expand, then your midriff, then your chest.
4. Breathe out slowly and let your attention rest on the breath's movement as the expansion leaves your chest, then your midriff, then your abdomen.

5. Let your shoulders and jaw release any tension and keep your attention on your abdomen and chest as you breathe in and out.

6. Close your eyes, if doing so comes naturally, and let yourself enjoy your breathing.

Next is a similar mindful breathing technique that you can use as often as you like. This exercise will work on your breathing muscles—the diaphragm—and make them more flexible and strong, providing a deeper and fuller breath. (This exercise is also available at http://www.newharbinger .com/41283.)

EXERCISE: PROLONGED EXHALATION

In this exercise you will practice exhaling slowly through your nostrils. Done as slowly as possible, this will lower your heart rate and help you wind down. It's helpful to direct your attention toward your throat. By slightly constricting the muscles around your larynx, you can decrease the outgoing airflow, prolonging the exhalation. A real-world parallel is constricting the outgoing water flow from a hose by slightly squeezing the opening with your fingers. These are the same muscles you use when you fog up a pair of glasses with your breath, exhaling with a slightly hissing sound: "Haaah." For optimal results, after you lie down, place a pillow on your stomach; this makes it easier to feel the movements of your abdomen when you breathe.

1. Lie down on the floor; if it's a hard surface, you can use a camping pad or yoga mat for comfort. Keeping your mouth closed, take conscious control of your breathing and notice the air filling your lungs and expanding your whole belly. Notice that you are inviting a deep, slow breathing. Feel the pillow on your stomach moving up and down as you breathe. To help you regulate your breathing, imagine smelling something very pleasant. What would your breathing be like then?

2. After a minute or so, try slowly, gently prolonging the exhalation.

3. Take a deep breath and notice it lifting your abdomen. Exhale as slowly as you can, while noticing your body is grounded and still.

4. Repeat this for two minutes before returning to your regular breathing.

BEING HERE AND NOW: A CONTINUOUS TRAINING OF THE MIND

We've given you lots of exercises so that you can find the ones that suit you best. We encourage you to visit the "mindfulness gym" throughout this program. We suggest you choose one exercise that you can do daily and one of our recorded guided audio exercises. (You'll find all of them at http:// www.newharbinger.com/41283.)

We recommend you try out "The Breathing Anchor" and "Body Scan." These popular exercises are common fundamentals of any mindfulness training. Another popular exercise is "Me, Here, Now, as Sturdy as an Oak."

TAKING ACTION: WHAT YOU CAN DO BEFORE READING THE NEXT CHAPTER

Here are some activities we suggest you do before moving on to the next chapter. First, look back at how you rated your life in your Life Compass at the beginning of this chapter. Is there anything you want to do more or less of and can schedule into your week? How can you use mindfulness to help you identify, plan, and carry out these activities?

- **Embrace a value.** Make time for taking at least one concrete action toward one of the life values you identified previously.

- **Recharging.** Schedule at least two restorative activities that also reflect values you have not pursued lately. Try to use one mindfulness activity in going about your daily routine.

- **Mindfulness.** Choose one exercise to do in daily life (on the go) and choose one guided audio exercise from http://www.newharbinger.com/41283.

When doing these activities, see if you can approach them with a mindful attitude—that is, as nonreactively, as nonjudgmentally, and as openheartedly as possible—even to the more challenging thoughts and feelings that might show up. In Chapter 5 we will guide you even further into what we call "willingness" as a stance to take with challenging feelings.

FOLLOW JOHN AND ANGELA IN THEIR EFFORTS TO LIVE A MORE MEANINGFUL AND BALANCED LIFE

John

Recharging

I've planned to meet Mia and just hang out and not do anything special. Maybe we'll make dinner together. Then on Sunday I'll go to a café and have breakfast with a good book.

Mindfulness

I was thinking of doing the "Breathing Anchor" exercise twice at lunch this week.

Everyday mindfulness: *I like the sound of this, in that it doesn't take up time. I'll be mindful when I drive to work every day and note how my body moves with the movement of the car.*

CHAPTER 3 EXPANDED SECTION

In this expanded section we'll cover these topics:

- Mindfulness and the judging mind

- Challenges when practicing mindfulness

Mindfulness Can Help Us Spot the Reactive and Judging Mind We Automatically Use

Even if we have "everything"—a happy childhood, good looks, a loving partner, wonderful children, and money in the bank—we still feel pain, partly because painful things happen to *all* of us sooner or later, partly because we ourselves create pain by how we assign value to things, or judge them. The habitual reactive mind is inclined to judge situations. We can always find examples of other people we see as better looking, happier, richer, or more successful.

One way to keep closer tabs on our continual judging is to differentiate between *facts* and *value judgments*. Let's start with a simple illustration. Imagine a pen—a normal, plastic pen. Its actual properties are that it's made of plastic, metal, and ink. These are facts. If you now look at the pen and think to yourself, "This pen looks cheap," you've applied a value judgment to the pen. The pen itself is neither cheap nor exclusive; it's just made of plastic, metal, and ink. But your mind has attached a certain note or tone to it that comes from your mind, and not from the real facts of the pen. Now, if we imagine that for some reason the entire human population were wiped out one morning, would the pen still consist of plastic, metal, and ink? Yes, it would. Would it seem cheap? No, because there'd be no one around to judge the looks of the pen.

It can be trickier to distinguish between facts and value statements when it comes to value statements about ourselves. We give examples in the table, "Common Painful Value Statements."

Similarly, we can pass judgment on ourselves. As the judgment feels true, we take it as a truth, and we miss the phenomenon that has happened: a judgment from the mind, not a fact or inherent characteristic of ourselves. It's not easy to distinguish between facts and judgments, and the brain can always find "proof" that what we think is "really true."

There are some particularly common painful themes that our minds keep telling us; we've listed some of them in the table. If we take these thoughts to be true, they can torment us. So how shall we deal with them? One way out that many people spontaneously take is to "think positive"—because isn't it just a matter of swapping bad thoughts for good ones?

Common Painful Value Statements

Theme	Example
Alienation	"I'm not like everyone else." "No one understands me." "There's something seriously wrong with me."
Belittling	"I'm less important than others." "I bring nothing to this world." "I give my loved ones nothing."
Moral weakness	"I'm a person with low moral standards." "I'm disgusting and repulsive." "If only you knew what I've done." "If only you knew the terrible thoughts I've had."
Lack of willpower/work ethic	"I can't do anything." "I'm totally useless." "I'm lazy." "I've got no self-control."
Hopelessness/helplessness	"Things will never get better." "I'll never make it." "Life's meaningless." "I'm a broken person."
Incompetence	"I'm a phony." "I'm useless at everything." "People will soon see through me."
Failure	"I deserve this." "This is all my fault." "If people knew the real me, they wouldn't like me."
Unreliability	"I can't be trusted." "I always let people down."

Of course, we can practice thinking positively; at least it will help build mental flexibility! But there are problems with "thinking positive." As soon as we think of something "positive," it puts us in contact with the "negative." It's just how the brain works. Say that you think you're incompetent, and you want to prove yourself wrong and convince yourself that you are, in fact, competent. You might start by thinking about a time when you did something really well and felt like a success. The brain, which is effectively hardwired to associate opposites, then automatically starts to remind you of other occasions when you failed. When we think in terms of "positive" or "negative," "good" or "bad," "better than" or "worse than," we are assigning a value to what we do and to ourselves and others. For an approach that is both mindful and wise, try the following:

- When your brain judges or labels reality, do nothing other than curiously notice. Do not try to find any reasons for the truth value of this judgment.

- Put the label "judging" onto the judgment (silently, in your head) and try lovingly patting your cheek with a soft hand when you notice this (as a loving and wise grandmother would have done). This can help you not get caught in another judgment about having a judgment. Actually, you can try this out right now!

- Tell yourself, "I deserve love simply by virtue of being who I am." We are who we are, and this statement lies beyond the various labels we attach to ourselves.

This final claim—"I deserve love simply by virtue of being who I am"—can arouse irritation or trigger thoughts intended to prove the contrary. The brain automatically elicits the counter-thought "I don't deserve love." What we're looking for here is more specifically "simply by virtue of being who I am." We maintain that you're worthy of love, both from others and from yourself, simply because you are you. Your value has nothing to do with your achievements or lack thereof. We are each unique, boundless, valuable, and beautiful in our own way. And this is true of you, even if your mind finds it hard to believe right now.

You're worthy of the love of others and yourself. This is true no matter what they, or you, think about what you do, have done, or look like. You deserve love for no other reason than that you are who you are, which goes beyond all the labels we attach to ourselves.

A growing body of work shows that self-empathy is healthy (for example, Breines et al., 2014; Germer & Neff, 2013; Baer, Lykins & Peters, 2012; Albertson, Neff, & Dill-Shackleford, 2014; Allen & Leary, 2010; Smeets, Neff, Alberts, & Peters, 2014; Kearney et al., 2013; Abaci & Arda, 2013; Heernan, Grin, McNulty, & Fitzpatrick, 2010; Neff, 2010; Neff, 2012). Showing ourselves kindness is good for us (we will expand on the subject of being kind to ourselves in Chapter 8).

Common Challenges with Mindfulness Exercises

Though practicing mindfulness is pretty simple and straightforward, we usually get questions from the people we teach it to. Here are some of the most common, with our answers.

I can't concentrate.

It's not at all strange that you lose focus and your thoughts sail away. The brain is hardwired to make associations and attend to something new. The good news is that every time you notice your thoughts are elsewhere, you're actually being mindful. Sometimes we try to focus and concentrate so much that we tense up and end up struggling—the opposite of the effect we are after. You're not in competition with yourself or engaged in some kind of struggle; you can let yourself "land" in the present moment or relax into it. It's more a matter of letting go than of achieving.

It feels uncomfortable and I can't relax.

Mindfulness is not synonymous with relaxation. It's about being aware of what you're experiencing in the here and now. A consequence of mindfulness might well be that you feel more relaxed, but you could also realize how tense and stressed you are. When you press the stop button and focus on how you're feeling, you may connect with tensions you were previously unaware of. If you've spent a lot of time trying to distract yourself from or avoid distressing thoughts and feelings, it's natural that you'll feel the heat when you apply the brakes. You might not like it at the time, but ultimately it's healthy and healing.

I fall asleep. Why?

We're used to shifting focus from one sense to another, from one stimulus to another. When we practice mindfulness, we're trying to focus on one thing at a time, and this can make us drowsy. Closed eyes also tend to be associated with rest or sleep.

If you get too little sleep during the week, and while practicing mindfulness you feel like dropping off, this will alert you to your sleep deficit. But not to worry; this is very common at first. The more you practice mindfulness, the less likely you are to fall asleep. If you start to feel sleepy, open your eyes, or if you are sitting, stand up.

I don't have time to do the exercises! There are a thousand other things I should be doing.

It's common for people to have trouble practicing mindfulness because they're thinking about all the things they "should" be doing instead of sitting passively listening to an exercise. If this is you, then these exercises are probably just what the proverbial doctor ordered! See if you can allow yourself some "me time" instead of getting diverted to all the musts. Can you view your mindfulness exercise as a little treat, or a bit of exercise for your well-being? Make sure your exercise surroundings are as serene as possible. You could even light some candles, add fresh flowers or a blooming plant, or do something else that you find soothing to make it feel calm and stress-free.

You've made it through Chapter 3—high five! And we hope you have planted several seeds of mindfulness to water in the coming weeks. In the next chapter you will learn a simple strategy to start making beneficial changes to manage stress in your life.

Change Your Life to Make It More Meaningful and Less Stressful

Man is not the sum of what he has already, but rather the sum of what he does not yet have, of what he could have.

—Jean Paul Sartre

ACT involves accepting what you can't change. You may recall that the A in ACT stands for *acceptance*, and we'll discuss that in depth in the next chapter. But the C in ACT is just as important. It stands for the *commitment* you make to make changes that move your life in a meaningful and values-driven direction. This chapter is about what you can actually do to change a situation that is not working. We'll show you efficient ways to bring about that change—you'll learn practical problem-solving methods to take on tough situations and circumstances. You may find these simple methods surprisingly life changing. We'll also dive into an important topic when it comes to managing stress: moving your body.

Before we begin, we'd like you to take a look at the past week and repeat a few key insights from the preceding chapter. Then we'll introduce you to a new tool to give you a better view of how you live your life. We'll also follow up on how you did on your other activities.

SO HOW ARE YOU DOING?

Answer the following questions and rate how effective each recovery activity was on a scale of 0 (no recovery) to 10 (significant recovery).

Activity	Completed?			Recovery, 0 to 10?
Took a small step on the basis of a value	Yes	Partly	No	
Practiced mindfulness at least once	Yes	Partly	No	
Did at least one recovery activity	Yes	Partly	No	

External Events That Got in the Way

If you replied "No" to any of the questions, write down any external events that got in the way of your completing the activity. How could you overcome such obstacles in the future?

Activity	External obstacle	Ideas on how I can deal with this
Took a small step on the basis of a value		
Practiced mindfulness at least once		
Did at least one recovery activity		

Internal Responses That Showed Up

Write down any negative thoughts, emotions, or physical sensations that arose and how you addressed them when doing your exercises, mindfulness sessions, short breaks, or new sleeping habits.

Activity	Internal responses (feelings, thoughts, bodily sensations)	How did you address these? (By avoiding, with mindfulness, other?)
Took a small step on the basis of a value		
Practiced mindfulness at least once		
Did at least one recovery activity		

KEY POINTS FROM CHAPTER 3

Mindfulness helps you stay focused and open. Many of us live in a culture where information processing is at the center of most days. We have gotten so used to using our thinking that we sometimes forget we have five other senses: touching, smelling, hearing, seeing, and tasting. Dwelling excessively in thoughts about the past or future can add to your overall stress level, and you can miss out on what is happening here and now. By practicing mindfulness in daily life and doing guided exercises, you can develop the habit of staying open to what you are feeling inside and nonjudgmental, focusing on the here and now.

How Have You Been Embracing Your Values?

Now let's go back to the tool for monitoring how you live your life, introduced in the previous chapter: the Life Compass.

What does your Life Compass look like for the past week? Think about each area and fill in a score.

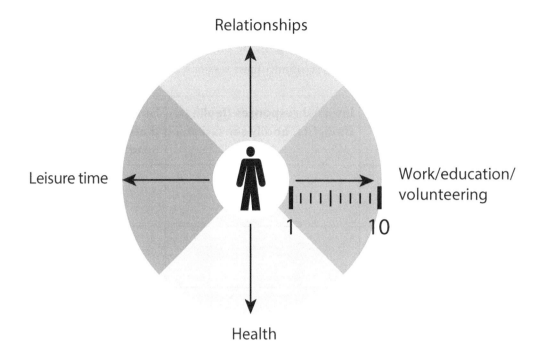

Relationships

Leisure time

Work/education/
volunteering

1   10

Health

Remember, the score you give is completely subjective; you base it solely on your own personal circumstances and limitations. Bear in mind both quantity and quality. It might be helpful to have your already completed compass in front of you. (If you don't want to write in this book, you can download blank compass forms at http://www.newharbinger.com/41283.)

Don't worry if your scoring in the four compass areas is uneven. It's perfectly normal not to always have a nice round circle. Different areas demand our attention from week to week, but if the imbalance persists you might want to ask yourself how you are living your life. Perhaps it's time to change something? With your Life Compass ratings in mind, is there anything you'd want to do more or less of over the coming week? Some area you'd like to give more priority to? It's best to choose a small action that you think you'll be able to manage.

_____

_____

_____

_____

CORE SECTION: CHANGE WHAT IS NOT WORKING

We encounter a lot of difficult, distressing, and painful events in our lives, and often we have no choice but to accept the difficult internal responses that they trigger in us. But we can change or prevent some of these unwanted events from occurring. This chapter is about identifying what stresses you and starting to see what you can do to improve your situation. We'll also be mapping out, step by step, how you can achieve such changes.

These changes don't have to be drastic. Indeed, sometimes just tweaking your actions to align slightly better with your values can be enough to make a significant difference over time. In a later part of the chapter we'll explore the amazing benefits of physical exercise.

Problem Solving in the Face of Stress

As a species, we are phenomenal at reasoning and problem solving; in fact, we're so smart that we've even made it to the moon. So our brains are already experts at problem solving. But sometimes we're not so sure of ourselves, perhaps because we've once been bitten or we dislike certain types of changes. Unhelpful thoughts may pop into our head, such as "I know I could ask for help, but I may look stupid or unprofessional. What if she thinks I'm being pushy?" In later chapters we'll be talking more about how you can handle such troubling thoughts and feelings, but we hope that you can already take on the challenge of changing something that's stressing you, when working toward what you value in your life. We'll be guiding you through some methods that research tells us are most effective for solving problems (e.g., Fantin, 2014; Cornell, 2010; Novick & Bassok, 2005; Wang & Chiew, 2010; Öllinger, Jones, & Knoblich, 2008; Mayer, 1992). We'll ask you to choose a problem that you can start to solve in the coming week or two. It's okay if the problem is a big one; you can start with intermediate steps or milestone solutions. The important thing is taking the first step.

EXERCISE: PROBLEM SOLVING, STEP BY STEP

1. **Define the problem**

   A problem properly clarified is a problem half solved. An important step in problem solving is therefore to spend time stating your problem as concretely as you can. Say, for instance, that you've noticed that you feel inadequate. Describing the problem as "I feel inadequate" is vague and abstract. A more specific description will give you a more precise understanding of what triggers such feelings, such as "I can't focus on my job because I keep getting interrupted." This more concrete description of *what is actually happening* can help you come up with actual solutions.

   Shortly we will ask you to start by choosing something you want to change. Again, at this stage it's good to choose something you can try out before moving on to the next chapter. If your problem is a big one, break it down into smaller subproblems that you can solve one piece at a time.

Maybe you think that someone else is the problem, and that might well be the case. But it's easy to fall into the cognitive trap that everything will be fine as soon as that other person changes. You have little or no control over how other people behave, even if sometimes you wish you did. What you *do* have full control over is how you act yourself. So the most effective course of action is to focus on what *you* can do.

There are also times when you might feel that the problem is beyond your direct control, such as when you encounter a difficult life situation: you are diagnosed with a serious disease, or you experience the death of a relative. We don't mean to minimize your problems, but what's happened has happened, and there's nothing anyone can do about it. Disease, death, and other unavoidable life events are best met by accepting the emotions they trigger, as we will discuss in the next chapter.

Even if the cause of our problem is something we must live with, there's often a little wiggle room for us to apply problem-solving techniques and bring about change. Even if we're face to face with death, we may have some choice in how we experience our remaining time on earth.

If something seriously distressing has happened, such as abuse, there's nothing we can do about the event itself—but we can learn to live with the painful aspects of the event in ways that do not cause us additional harm.

First, let's see what John did at this stage of the process:

Which area are you experiencing as most stressful right now: leisure time, health, work/education, or relationships?

Work

Describe one of the things that you find problematic.

I'm stressed out at work.

Can you elaborate and describe even more concretely?

I don't have time to do all the things I need to do, and I feel that I'm constantly behind in my work.

What are the possible causes of this problem?

I'm team leader for two teams. Everyone else has no more than one team to work with.

Define your problem in as clear and concrete terms as possible:

I'm team leader for one team too many, which means that I don't have the time to do what I'm supposed to do.

Now it's your turn.

Which area are you experiencing as most stressful right now: leisure time, health, work/education, or relationships?

_____

_____

Describe one of the things that you find problematic.

_____

_____

_____

_____

Can you elaborate and describe even more concretely?

_____

_____

_____

_____

What are the possible causes of this problem?

_____

_____

_____

_____

Define your problem in as clear and concrete terms as possible:

_____

_____

_____

_____

2.   Elicit solutions through brainstorming

What can really interrupt a creative process is our occasional tendency to dismiss solutions through hasty critical evaluations before we've even had time to think them through. Sometimes it's as if we get stuck and unable to do anything about the situation. But often there's at least one solution to run with; the trick is to spot it. Brainstorming can help us do just that. Brainstorming is about collecting as many ideas as we can, and by refraining from passing judgment before we consider *all* solutions—be they crazy, funny, serious, or clever—we can find new, previously unconsidered ways to solve a problem.

Now it's time for you to give it a go—write down all the solutions you can think of. A little time pressure often helps, so if you have a clock or a watch handy, give yourself five minutes. The more possibilities you come up with, the more likely you are to spot a workable solution.

But before you start, look at the possible solutions that John brainstormed:

- *Talk to my boss*

- *Change jobs*

- *Blow the place up*

- *Work more hours*

- *Skip the team meetings*

- *Ask for a colleague to run the team with me*

- *Ask for more pay*

- *Suggest that we stop working in teams*

- *Resign my role of team leader*

- *Merge the teams*

- *Fire all the members of one team*

Now it's your turn. Write down all the possible solutions you can think of.

My solutions: _____

_____

_____

_____

_____

_____

3. Evaluate the pros and cons of the different solutions

You now have a list of solutions with varying degrees of feasibility. The next step is to decide which would be most effective in bringing about the change you want to see. Factor into your ratings both the short- and long-term consequences of each solution. Blowing up your office is, to be sure, a very effective *short-term* solution to avoid having to work overtime, but in the *long term* it will only create a whole bunch of new problems (such as how to get along with your new cellmate).

Assign each solution a score of 0 to 10 depending on how helpful you think it would be in solving your problem. Write the score alongside each one. Several solutions can have the same score.

4. Select and schedule

By scheduling implementation of your chosen solutions, you increase the chances of the change actually becoming a reality. This also gives you an opportunity to think about possible impediments and how you can overcome them. The goal should not be an emotional one.

With an emotional goal, you strive for a certain feeling, such as "to feel secure," "to feel loved," or "to be happy." These feelings are important but generally cannot be achieved directly or by force of will. Emotions come and go—it's impossible to remain in a particular emotional state. Emotional goals, therefore, have failure built into them.

"Dead man's goals" are goals that a corpse would have a better chance of attaining than you, such as getting rid of feelings or not being in a certain state. A dead person is better than you are, for example, at relaxing, feeling no pain, and being unburdened by worry or guilt. Let's try to avoid those goals.

The goals we strongly recommend are specific, time-bound, quantifiable, and realistic.

- *Specific* goals are concrete and self-contained. A nonspecific goal might be "I want more time to myself." A specific—and better—formulation would be: "I'll take a walk twice a week at lunch."

- *Time-bound* means that the goal can be planned for a certain time. A non-time-bound goal might be "I'll talk to my boss about my workload." A time-bound goal would be "I'll talk to my boss about my workload after Thursday's meeting."

- *Quantifiable* means that the goal can be measured so that you can tell whether you've attained it. A non-quantifiable goal might be "I want to be a better colleague." A quantifiable goal would be "I want to meet my colleagues more often and have lunch with them at least once a week."

- *Realistic* goals are not too ambitious or unattainable and can be attained within a reasonable time period. An unrealistic goal for someone with a full-time job and young children might be "I'll train five times a week and have a nice, long uninterrupted breakfast every day." Unrealistic goals like this just lead to failure and encourage us to give up the idea of making goals altogether. A realistic goal would be "I'll train once a week and have a nice, unhurried breakfast at work with a colleague once a month."

This is what John planned:

My solution. Tell my boss my problem and ask for help prioritizing the teams.

1. Write a list of the different things I do with the team and what a team leader is expected to do.

2. Write down suggestions I want to put to my boss.

3. Schedule a meeting with my boss.

When will I do it? Next week after the team meeting.

What are the possible obstacles? That my boss isn't there. That there's no one available who can take over the role of team leader.

Solutions to the obstacles: Arrange a meeting in advance with my boss. Have a backup plan; suggest that someone else can eventually take over the team and that I can show them the ropes.

Will I tell anyone else what I'm doing? My friend Dennis.

Evaluation: It went well, although I could've explained more clearly what I need to do for me to enjoy my job and to develop my skills.

Now do the same thing with your suggested solution.

My solution _____

_____

_____

_____

If you want to break the solution down into steps, you can do so here.

1. _____

_____

_____

_____

2. _____

_____

_____

_____

3. _____

_____

_____

_____

When will I do it? _____

_____

_____

_____

What are the possible obstacles? _____

_____

_____

_____

Solutions to the obstacles: _____

_____

_____

_____

Will I tell anyone else what I'm doing? _____

_____

_____

_____

As you bring a solution, or several, to mind, we encourage you to schedule it in your calendar. If it would be helpful, set a reminder—or you could also picture someone who inspires you and gives you courage, and let that person serve as a role model for you, imagining the person is walking together with you on your path of bold change. Maybe even keep a picture of this person somewhere visible.

5. Evaluation

The final stage of the problem-solving model is to evaluate how well it went. If you've already tried your solution, know that we'll come back to it in the beginning of Chapter 5 to find out how you did. See the solution as an exciting experiment, and remain open-minded about the possible outcome.

In the second part of this chapter we devote our attention to a critically important topic when it comes to stress management: moving the body. Moving your body can help reduce your stress, and it can also help you realize your value of being healthy.

Physical Exercise—Your Mind and Body Are One, So Exercise Both

Did you ever go for a run and later that same day you were astonished at how amazingly regenerated you felt? There was no magic to it—or actually, there was! When we exercise, the body secretes endorphins (hormones that give us a sense of well-being), and levels of the stress hormone cortisol are normalized. Exercise gives a good boost to the immune system and can prevent harmful stress hormones from reaching the brain (Liston, McEwen, & Casey, 2009; Segerstrom & Miller, 2004). It also helps counteract a number of other problems, such as insomnia, depression, and chronic anxiety (e.g., Ehrman, Gordon, Visich, & Keteyian, 2008; Cooney et al., 2013; Rethorst & Madhukar, 2013; Cotman, Berchtold, & Christie, 2007; Dunn et al., 2005; Gleeson et al., 2011). In this program, exercise is a core component of recharging your life, body, and soul, and we cannot stress too much the benefits of making your body move, both to strengthen your body to counteract harmful stress, and to create the energy and health needed for meaningful actions.

However, there are a few cautions. First, you can overexercise and wear your body out if you don't take time to rest. If you push yourself to the limit every day, consider resting your body instead. Second, some use exercise to avoid distressing feelings and thoughts. If this is the main reason you exercise, it can merely perpetuate the troubles you're avoiding, rather than dealing with them. (In Chapter 6, we'll unpack how this kind of avoidance can cause further problems.) If you're suffering from burnout, we don't recommend attempting intense exercise; start with gentler activities—a twenty-minute walk rather than a session at the gym. (You'll find more information on burnout in a bonus chapter at http://www.newharbinger.com/41283.) Consult your doctor if you have questions about the optimal level of exercise for you.

EXERCISE: WORKING TOWARD A HEALTHY BODY WILL ALSO IMPROVE YOUR MIND

We each have our own preferences for moving our bodies. Some have a regular workout routine and maybe even an identity as a "sports person"; for others, it's a major effort to just go for a walk. Still others may have lost their routine—or never even had one. We're all different, and wherever you are, it's never too late to start walking the walk. As we encourage you to take steps toward nurturing your body with exercise and movement, old friends (your thoughts) might rear their heads, saying you shouldn't, or can't, or that you're too out of shape, or that you can never be as fit as before, or as fit as someone else. If you encounter these thoughts, we encourage you to not try to argue with them, but simply bring them along to your workout.

First, we invite you to explore your values concerning health and exercise. Why might this be important to you? What values could inspire you to move in this direction? How could a healthy body help you live the values you have in other areas of your life? When you are ninety, looking back at your life, what kind of relationship to your body and exercise would you like to have had?

_____

_____

_____

_____

To beat stress and keep up good health, we recommend both a daily and a weekly routine of moving your body.

Daily Routine Exercise

Here are some ways people include movement in their daily routine:

- Going for a walk

- Getting off the bus one stop earlier when going to work, or parking the car a bit farther away and walking to the office

- Standing up from the office chair and stretching every half hour

- Choosing to walk to the grocery store instead of taking transit

- Using stairs instead of the elevator

- Commuting by bike, or using the bike for errands

What concrete actions, in line with your values, could you start taking? We recommend including at least twenty to thirty minutes of moderate activity in your daily routine. Choose a couple of routines that would be easiest for you to follow through on. Write down what you prefer as a daily routine:

_____

_____

Add these to your calendar or smartphone and maybe put up a reminder note to yourself if you find that helpful.

Intense Exercise

Here are some ways people like to do more intense exercise:

- Walking

- Yoga

- Jogging

- Swimming

- Running

- Dance class

- Martial arts

- Biking

- Housework

- Gardening

- Working out at the gym (weights, aerobic machines, classes)

We recommend that you schedule one or two sessions a week in which you are physically active and raise your heart rate for at least half an hour; whether you go to the gym, jog, or go for a brisk walk, the important thing is to get your pulse up. If you find yourself in a condition where this is difficult—for example, you have a long commute or small children to take care of—then choose whatever level of exercise you can fit in, and see if you can add at least one thirty-minute brisk walk a week as a start.

Write down what you prefer as intense exercise; choose activities that you can actually follow through with, and schedule them on your calendar. You can also track your exercise after you've done it, marking the day with a star, heart, highlighting, or other indicator—or an X if you didn't manage it. At month's end, see how many days got the mark of exercise.

_____

_____

_____

TAKING ACTION: WHAT YOU CAN DO BEFORE READING THE NEXT CHAPTER

Schedule a day for reading Chapter 5. About a week from now would be good. Make a note on your calendar or set an alarm on your phone.

You can also look back at how you rated your life in your Life Compass at the beginning of this chapter. Is there anything you want to do more or less of and can schedule? Then continue with the following:

- *Solve a problem.* Address the solution you've chosen for the problem that's making you stressed.

- *Recovery.* Schedule at least one recovery activity and do it.

- *Exercise.* Schedule one or two (or more) pulse-raising exercise sessions (at minimum, a brisk thirty-minute walk) and establish or continue a daily routine of moving your body.

- *Mindfulness exercise.* Schedule and carry out at least one mindfulness exercise before reading the next chapter. Also, do your best to stay open and nonjudgmental to any negative internal response that shows up when you're doing your activities during the week. See if you can bring curiosity to all that is going on inside of you.

FOLLOW JOHN AND ANGELA IN THEIR EFFORTS TO LIVE A MORE MEANINGFUL AND BALANCED LIFE

John

Problem solving

I've decided to arrange a time to go see my boss to ask if he can help me prioritize tasks related to the teams and duties I'm currently managing.

Recovery

I've arranged to meet Mia to go to an exhibition and have dinner on Friday. I've also decided to cancel work that I was planning to do Sunday evening. I'm going to book an hour's massage this week.

Exercise

I'll continue cycling to work every day. I'll also go for a ride in the woods on Wednesday and a jog on Monday.

Mindfulness

I've set aside time to do the "Body Scanning" guided mindfulness exercise on Wednesday. I'll do the "Breathing Anchor" during lunch on Tuesday.

If you want to learn more about how to get "unstuck" from stressful habits or find out more about how to deal with difficult choices, the expanded section of this book is for you.

CHAPTER 4 EXPANDED SECTION

In this expanded section of the chapter we will cover how to create more flexibility in our lives and how to deal with difficult choices.

Do the Opposite—and Create Flexibility

As we go through life, we all have psychological issues to struggle with, our own Achilles' heel. It's common to go through periods of restlessness or insomnia. And statistics show that many people will find themselves at risk for abusing alcohol, if they are not already. We may go through periods of anxiety, obsessive-compulsive behavior, and feeling low and sad at one time or another; some of us will become so troubled that we meet the criteria for clinical depression or clinical anxiety in some way.

If we're very stressed for a long time, these old habits of mind and behavior might show up again. Panic attacks and depressive moods are the most common symptoms of chronic stress, and stress can exacerbate any tendencies we might have toward alcohol abuse, compulsiveness, or other such troublesome behaviors. It can even be a slippery slope toward more serious problems (such as anxiety disorders and major depression). Indeed, you may find yourself feeling you need to seek professional help.

The best approach, of course, is to manage your problems so that they don't get out of hand, and the key to doing this is to be aware of your psychological health, so if it becomes too out of balance you know that you have been too stressed for too long and need to recover. We each have our own signs of being off-kilter, and you probably know yours, based on past experiences. Maybe you've noticed that you're inclined to turn to the bottle or are prone to panic attacks, insomnia, depression, rigidity, or angry defensiveness when you become too stressed. When we notice ourselves struggling with these problems, it's worth trying to do the opposite of what you've been doing to cope. This can create flexibility and help you break unhealthy patterns (more about that soon).

What happens to you when you're stressed for long periods? Do you notice any typical patterns of behavior? Are there things that you do more or less of? In the following table, you may recognize some of the things people commonly do when stressed from Chapter 1. If you don't see one or more of your own behaviors here, add them in the blanks that follow.

Become controlling, rigid	Do too much of everything	Stop doing customary things
Eat a lot more or less	Become obsessed with sex	Arrive late at meetings
Consume too much alcohol (or other drugs)	Strive for efficiency	Sleep a lot more
Avoid others	Do things too quickly	Shop too much

Give myself less time to sleep	Stop asking for help	Become argumentative, short with people
Insist on perfection	Stop listening to others	Take on too much responsibility
Ignore other people's feelings; force others to do my will	Stop taking breaks	Sleep less

What coping behaviors of your own can you add to this list?

_____

_____

_____

DOING "THE OPPOSITE"

Does your choice of action go on autopilot when you are stressed?

By becoming aware of your automatic responses and challenging them, you can become more flexible in the dance of life and create more action space for yourself. Now think of something you do when you're stressed (like wolfing down your dinner) that you want to challenge.

What does your stressful behavior look like? _____

_____

_____

Is it connected to any value? _____

Now we challenge you to do the opposite, or at least try a different approach, to stretch your behavior a bit. By doing the opposite, two exciting things might happen:

You learn that it's not the end of the world, and that you're free to act in new ways. If you always prepare a report or a presentation at work meticulously, try making an easygoing effort next time. (We don't mean doing a horrible job on a presentation, just not stressing to make it *perfect*: "good enough" can be the opposite of "perfect" in this case.) Doing a perfect job might be a life value and is not wrong per se; the problems start when you feel forced to always do something in a certain way. By doing the opposite, you can give yourself an immediate and healthy experience of "surviving" or being good enough as you are—even if the outcome lacks your usual perfection.

Your autopilot won't switch on in the same way, and you'll have to be more mindful. Have you ever had the feeling that your life is on autopilot, that you're somehow remote controlled? That you've arrived at work without really recalling how you got there? Or that everything you do feels routine and that nothing new happens? Much of what we do often or habitually feels like this. But when we start consciously doing the opposite of our usual, the autopilot is disengaged. Finding ourselves in an unfamiliar situation and unaccustomed to acting in a particular way may make us more mindful of our existence in the here and now.

Write down in the space provided one or more examples of behavior that challenges your stressful habits. You're the expert on yourself, so you know what's appropriate for you. Whatever you take on, make sure it won't be too difficult for you to do (or not do!) and that it feels important, even a little thrilling. Describe in detail your usual automatic response and what you plan to do "opposite" instead.

If you have a hard time knowing what your stressful behaviors are, ask a friend, partner, or family member; they will probably give you an honest answer.

Stressful behavior	Opposite behavior

John's Example

I reckon I'm a bit obsessed with working out and feel guilty every time I stop going to the gym regularly. I can feel stressed about not having time to train. My life rule is: "I must have a good body and be fit." I'll try not going to the gym at all this week and eating whatever I like.

The following section is dedicated to the stress we can find ourselves in when dealing with a dilemma in life. If you're facing a dilemma right now, our advice may be especially worth trying out.

When Difficult Choices Become Obstacles

Difficult choices can be really stressful. To resolve the dilemma, we often stop and try to find the best solution by thinking through possible consequences and scenarios. Sometimes this helps, but other times we can get tangled up in our thoughts and can't make a decision. It can feel like we've run aground; the inertia this causes fills us with an almost paralyzing sense of confusion and anxiety.

Such ambivalence can be powerfully stress-inducing, especially if it concerns important decisions about a relationship or a job.

The choices we make in life are rarely self-evident or clear-cut; we rarely know what a decision will lead to, and we rarely have full control over what will actually happen. But the brain wants to believe there's a right choice and a wrong one, that "all I have to do is the right thing and I'll be happy." So the brain does its utmost to predict the consequences of one possibility or another.

We may search our mind so hard for the right choice that we end up in a kind of cognitive loop, and our brain crashes; we end up unable to decide or to direct our energy, and ultimately we fail to act.

Examples of difficult stress-inducing decisions:

- To remain in or end a relationship

- To raise a sensitive matter with a partner

- To apply for a course or do a degree

- To take on more responsibility at work

- To take on less responsibility at work

- To work more hours

- To work fewer hours

- To remain in or change a job

- To change a career

- To move to another town

- To move to another home

- To start a family or not

Are you facing any difficult decisions? Write them down here.

My difficult decisions _____

_____

_____

Our colleague, Dr. Russ Harris, offers lots of advice and information about dealing with difficult decisions:

- There are no easy answers. If only one alternative were much better than the other, the choice probably wouldn't be difficult. Allow space for the frustration—it's completely normal in this situation.

- Rome wasn't built in a day. Difficult decisions take time.

- No matter what you decide, you'll probably be nagged by doubt, worry, or anxiety. Can you allow these thoughts and feelings to exist without attaching any real importance to them?

- You always make choices. Not acting is also a choice. Not choosing is a psychological impossibility, and it's good to be aware of that. All choices have ramifications, both positive and negative.

If you're stuck in a difficult dilemma that consumes a lot of time and energy, here are some practical methods you can try daily for as long as you feel stuck:

Every Morning

- *Confirm the choice you make that day.* It can feel good to affirm the choice you've made that day. If you've chosen not to change anything on this particular day, you can say to yourself, "Today my choice is to not make any change." If you decide to make a change, confirm to yourself that it is your choice for the day.

- *Where do I stand in all this?* It's also good to think about where you stand in this dilemma. Which of your values do you want to accompany you in this tough decision? What are the pros and cons of the choice you made for that day, given what is important to you?

During the Day

- *Give the dilemma a name.* Dilemmas often set our minds churning and can send us on a path of recurring anxiety with seemingly no escape. One way to get some distance from our ruminations is to imagine it is a story being told again and again as a film on a loop, say, or a radio play that keeps replaying. Title the story: "Career Dilemma," for example. When your mental mill starts grinding, say: "Right; I'm seeing/hearing the 'Career Dilemma' story again." (Maybe I'll make popcorn for it this time.)

■ *Try to exercise a little self-compassion.* Difficult dilemmas can persist for a long time— years, in the case of something like ending a relationship. See if you can exercise a little self-compassion at this difficult time. Is there anything you can do to be kind to yourself?

It might help to put your situation down in writing. Describe it here:

If this dilemma had a name or title, it'd be: _____

My choice today is to _____

_____

_____

_____

How do I want act in this situation? What values are relevant to me here? _____

_____

_____

_____

What are the pros and cons of the choice I made for today, given what's important to me?

Pros: _____

_____

_____

_____

Cons: _____

_____

_____

_____

If I want to show myself some kindness in this difficult situation, I can do this: _____

_____

_____

_____

The Power of Structured Problem Solving and Exercise

We hope you've found methods in this chapter that will help you overcome obstacles in your everyday life. Taking a structured approach to problem solving has been tremendously helpful for us authors, both in work with clients and in our own lives. With a structured approach, a situation that seems confusing, overwhelming, and impossible to manage can, surprisingly often, become pretty clear. We can overcome quite a few of life's obstacles if we put our mind to it and make the choices that need to be made. As for physical exercise—well, it's pure magic, as long as you keep it at a healthy level. The next chapter is about the things we *cannot* change—and how to best deal with them.

Willingness to Face the Inevitable

Life isn't about waiting for the storm to pass ... It's about learning to dance in the rain.

—Vivian Greene

A spirit of willingness allows us to approach our difficult thoughts and feelings and the overall stress that may emerge when we confront people, situations, events, and other aspects of life that we cannot change. Indeed, we cannot successfully avoid our own stressful thoughts and feelings without creating a narrow life. When life becomes narrow, it can seem less meaningful and vital, and if we turn to drugs and alcohol as an avoidance strategy for stressful emotions and thoughts, this can unintentionally create more stress—for example, if we end up losing a job or important relationships.

Of course, there are many aspects of our lives that we *can* change. When we have the opportunity to make those changes to attain meaningful goals that help us reduce stress, that is an ideal situation. As we will discuss, willingness can help us move through doubts and fears that often occur when making even those changes that we really want to make. The technique of mindfulness can also give us a perspective from which to see whether we can make a change, and if so, what costs that change will incur. If the cost is worth it, we can use willingness to find the courage to make any changes that may naturally evoke stress.

Before we examine these issues further, let's check how you've done since last week, repeat the key points from the last chapter, and take a look at your Life Compass.

SO HOW ARE YOU DOING?

We asked you to solve a problem (or part of a problem) by this chapter. Did you do what you'd planned to?

Completed?	Yes	Partly	No
Did your action solve the problem?	Yes	Partly	No

What, If Anything, Is the Next Step You'll Take Toward Dealing With This Problem?

If you didn't give yourself time to implement the solution that you came up with in the previous chapter, you may want to continue working with it; if you weren't happy with it, maybe you'd like to try a new one. Note here how you'd like to proceed.

_____

_____

_____

_____

How did you do on the other activities? Answer these questions and rate how restorative each activity was on a scale of 0 (no recovery) to 10 (plenty of recovery).

Activity	Completed?			Recovery, 0 to 10?
Did at least one recovery activity	Yes	Partly	No	
Exercised at least twice	Yes	Partly	No	
Practiced mindfulness at least once	Yes	Partly	No	

External Events That Got in the Way

If you answered "No" to any of these questions, please note any external events that got in the way of your completing the activity. How could you overcome these obstacles in the future?

Activity	External obstacle	Ideas for how I could deal with this
Recovery		
Exercise		
Mindfulness		

Internal Responses That Showed Up

Write down any challenging thoughts, emotions, or physical sensations that arose when doing your workouts, mindfulness sessions, and recovery activities, and how you addressed them. Also note which strategy helped you most in proceeding with your activities.

Activity	Internal responses (feelings, thoughts, bodily sensations)	How did you address these? (By avoiding, with mindfulness, or other?)
Recovery		
Exercise		
Mindfulness		

How Have You Been Embracing Your Values?

How many steps have you taken this past week in the different areas? Remember, your score is completely subjective; it's based solely on your own personal circumstances and limitations. Consider all the things you've identified as important in each area, bearing in mind both quantity and quality. It may be helpful to have your already completed compass in front of you. (You can download a blank compass at http://www.newharbinger.com/41283.)

What does your Life Compass look like for the past week?

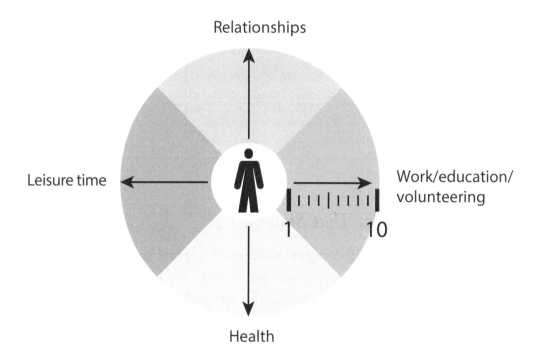

Again, don't worry if your attention to the different areas is uneven; that's perfectly normal and natural. Different areas will demand your attention from week to week, but if the imbalance persists you might want to ask yourself how you are living your life. Perhaps it's time to change something?

With your Life Compass rating in mind, is there anything you'd want to do more or less of over the coming week? Some area you'd like to give more priority to? It's best to choose a small action that you think you'll be able to manage.

_____

_____

_____

KEY POINTS FROM CHAPTER 4

Change is Often Possible

With a structured approach to problem solving, a situation that seems overwhelming and impossible to grasp can become pretty clear. We can overcome most of life's obstacles if we put our mind to it and look at them in a new way.

Move Your Body or Exercise to Reduce Stress

Exercise is one of the most efficient stress management techniques there is. A workout actually reduces the negative effect of stress hormones on the body and mind. Even short walks, or small movements such as standing up for a quick stretch, are good for your body. These small steps count, so don't discount them!

CORE SECTION: ENHANCING WILLINGNESS

We don't know what your life's like. But we authors—who are also experts on stress and how it's best handled—experience our own difficult, distressing, or painful moments. It's an intrinsic part of being human. Sometimes life's okay, wonderful even. Then something happens. You have too much to do at work. You fight with your partner. Your mother falls seriously ill, or your big brother's life falls apart.

This roller-coaster ride is normal for us as humans. Life has its ups and downs. We set ourselves unrealistic expectations if we think life should roll along smoothly and we should always feel good. Indeed, this only makes us depressed, angry, or sad when we don't typically feel as good as we think we *ought to*. These unrealistic and impossible assumptions about life can only send us on a downward spiral into misery. We begin to struggle with ourselves—and berate ourselves because life is tough.

There's a misconception in our society that life is meaningful only when everything's going well; when we're feeling bad, sad, tired, or bored, we get lured into believing that we're nothing but failures, living meaningless lives. The premise is that we have total control over life, so when things go wrong we have only ourselves to blame. If we appreciate life only when it's a bed of roses, we can easily become dissatisfied with a sizable part of our existence, because that sizable part is difficult and painful, no matter how "in control" we are. One of the founders of ACT, Professor Steven Hayes, expressed this well: "There's as much life in one moment of pain as in one moment of joy."

One cause for suffering is that we tend to compare our own worries, sadness, and emotional troubles with other people's polished exteriors (which look great!). We feel all the difficult, painful things going on inside us, convinced that other people are always doing better than we are, because externally they look fine, even great. (Just look at that happy family picture they posted on Facebook!) People seem so happy and contented, and their social media updates boast of their latest workouts, glorious travel adventures, happy children, and successful relationships. You've probably gone home after a really heavy day and asked yourself: "Why can't I be happy and contented and take life as it comes, like my friends and acquaintances do? They don't seem to be suffering from stress or anxiety or insomnia."

But here's the secret: they're suffering too. All of us feel pain and anxiety. No one who lives long enough can avoid the pain of having lost a loved one. Everyone experiences physical pain. Everyone experiences fear, anxiety, shame, grief, and bereavement. We all carry memories of embarrassing, humiliating, or distressing events. We all have our secret wounds. We might put on a happy, carefree mask and pretend that everything's fine, that life's a ball. But life isn't always so easy, and Prince Charming doesn't always show up at that ball. We often add to this naturally occurring pain by trying to avoid it or control it; this only leads to more pain.

To distinguish the parts of life that just happen from the things we actually have control over, here's how to differentiate what we call "natural stress" from "unnecessary stress."

Natural Stress

Life presents us all with natural stress. We fall ill, someone hurts us, we hurt ourselves, we fail, we sleep badly, we make fools of ourselves, and we feel lost and alone. This is natural, and not even the most sophisticated control and planning measures can give us immunity. Even if we tried to shelter ourselves from pain or illness, sooner or later life would still throw some hurdle or other in our way, and we'd be lonely and dissatisfied.

Someone we love will die. We'll get sick. And despite the many pleasures it brings, the love we feel for someone will break our hearts.

Natural stress, pain, or discomfort vary in strength; they range from irritation over some inconvenience to profound grief when a loved one dies. What follow are some of the common sources of stress that we encounter throughout our lives. And any emotional response we have to them—grief or anger, say—is completely natural, and we help ourselves by being open to these emotions.

Common Triggers of High Stress

Someone close to us dies. We'll all die, and people we love will die too.

Crises, personal and otherwise. We and our loved ones will end up in a crisis of some kind, be it relational, age-related, existential, whatever ("What do I want from life?" and "Who am I?").

Our past, our childhood. We all have our personal baggage, a heavy backpack of experiences to lug around. It's perfectly normal for our past to surface in the present in the form of painful, distressing, or embarrassing memories.

Pain. We all encounter physical and mental pain in our lives. Sometimes the pain is short-lived and sometimes it lasts a lifetime, but do we choose to stop living because of it?

Common Triggers of Moderate Stress

Disease, personal and otherwise. We'll all fall ill at times, as will the people we love.

Fatigue. Sometimes we're tired; other times we might feel chronically lethargic or weary from a lack of (quality) sleep.

Other people. We're all different, and certain other people are bound to rub us the wrong way—even people we love—when we have to see them every day.

Having to choose and decide. We must constantly make choices and decisions, some of which will lead to necessary pain in some way. Deciding not to decide is also a choice, but it is like choosing not to swim when you've been dropped in the middle of a lake—you may be saved or you may drown, but you have given up control of the situation.

Common Triggers of Minor Stress

Everyday events. These are familiar vexations like missing a bus or a train, accidentally dropping a plate or a glass, choosing what turns out to be the slowest checkout lane, or breaking something that will need fixing.

Avoiding Natural Stress Makes the Feelings and Situations Worse

What we call "unnecessary stress" is what we create by reacting to life's hurdles in unhelpful ways, such as when we deny, avoid, or struggle with the thoughts and feelings that life's hurdles create. We can become stressed about being stressed, anxious because we notice ourselves feeling sad, feel like a failure because we're afraid, and on and on we can go. When we don't allow ourselves to be humans—allowing ourselves to feel what we feel—we're defying nature; we're pretending we're Superman and can fly. When we judge ourselves because we feel a feeling that we are actually having, we are judging the wind because it is blowing, or the sun because it is shining. In other words, unnecessary stress is something we create when we don't allow natural stress to exist.

Imagine that you've broken your arm. What you feel is pure, natural pain. You can then let your thoughts run away with you: "I'm such a klutz! How stupid of me! And now I'll be out of work for months! What a disaster! I'll probably lose my job and won't ever find another one. I'm always so unlucky! It's so unfair!" These anticipated catastrophes create unnecessary stress and pain that does nothing to help the situation you're in and maybe even makes the broken arm hurt a little more; it also distracts you from more effectively fixing and recovering from the broken arm. The prudent thing to do is to acknowledge that it's happened and that it hurts—to be receptive to how it feels, to register the thoughts running through your mind; this is what the mindfulness training is for—and then to go to a doctor to get your arm x-rayed and put in a cast. This way you avoid layering unnecessary pain on top of the natural pain radiating from your broken arm in the here and now.

Being aware of when you overlay unnecessary stress onto natural stress can help you prevent your stress level from rising. A healthy attitude is to accept what's happened and to acknowledge the thoughts and feelings it naturally elicits. This will enable you to think more clearly and thus handle the situation in whatever way you think will help you the most in your life.

EXERCISE: THE HEALING HAND

"The Healing Hand" is a practical exercise in acceptance of the natural thoughts and feelings that you experience. It helps you tune in to what you're feeling and thinking, right here and right now. You can learn and then use this technique in whatever difficult situations life puts you in. The exercise comprises five steps that we suggest you try out for a total of three minutes. You can read the instructions, then set an alarm for three minutes or just look at a clock. But it's fine if you want to go on for longer. If you wish, you can also listen to these directions as a guided audio exercise at http://www.newharbinger.com/41283.

1. Find a quiet place to sit where you won't be disturbed for a while.

2. Think about an area in your life that's painful or difficult, or one you've been struggling with unsuccessfully for some time. Clarify your feelings and thoughts; let them be in you and settle in your body.

3. Place a hand on the part of your body where you feel these difficult emotions most acutely. Let your hand rest there for a while.

4. Say these three things to yourself:

   "This is a tough moment in my life."

   "Tough times are a part of life."

   "Someone, somewhere is also feeling the same tough thing right now."

5. See if you can let your tough emotions be in your body. You don't have to like them or want them—just let them be. Imagine your body opening up and making room for all of them.

6. Say to yourself: "May I hold my pain with kindness."

Common Questions about Emotions and Willingness

Psychologists often hear questions and comments like these. Perhaps you have similar thoughts running through your mind; knowing their commonality may help you feel you're not alone with them.

I can't cope with accepting all my emotions. If I do, I'll explode.

It's natural for powerful feelings to make us anxious, scared, or uncomfortable; it's equally natural for us to impulsively want to flee them. But our emotions can't harm us. Even the most intense emotions come and go in waves.

I have to get rid of these emotions so that I can start to live my life.

Trying to avoid or fight emotions is often counterproductive. In the short run, avoiding emotions can be helpful for coping with an acute situation, but in the long run it often stops us from living our lives. When we strive for important and meaningful things in life, what shows up is not only joy and excitement, but often fear of failure, rejection, and uncertainty. If we let these feelings steer us away from what we want, we might end up depressed or living a life we feel is not rewarding: "I'll wait until I feel better [emotionally], then I'll …" By waiting for the feeling to diminish, pass, or go away for good before we do what we want to do, we often put our life on hold—sometimes forever. The best strategy is often to approach our feelings, open up to them, and take steps in a valued direction. If you have severe and debilitating anxiety, we recommend you also talk to a therapist who uses a CBT approach.

My emotions are dangerous! They make me do crazy things.

There's usually a small interval of time between what we feel and what we then do—how we act on that emotion. If, when experiencing an intense emotion, we tend to react blindly in a way that isn't productive (a way that causes problems for us or someone else), we need to practice expanding this interval slightly. This makes it much easier for us to choose how to act on this emotion. One expansion method is to stop and take three deep breaths before deciding what to do.

Emotions: What Are They Good For?

There's a clear link between emotions and stress; when we're stressed, it can arouse patterns of emotions, and how we handle them in turn affects how stressed we get! It can become a bit of a vicious circle.

It's not uncommon for us to think that a happy life is a life free from negative emotions, so we reason that we should do all we can to avoid them. But this is a futile endeavor—emotions come to us whether we like it or not.

Emotions—even the negative ones—fulfill several functions. Most emotions are "negative" because they once conferred an evolutionary advantage in telling us to avoid threats and danger. You could say that an emotion is a messenger. It has something to tell us and activates a certain behavioral or cognitive pattern to help us manage different situations. Emotions aren't harmful; they are transient and can function as beacons that guide us through life. If you observe an imaging scanner's view of a person's brain reacting to an emotional stimulus, you'll see that an emotional response, regardless of how strong it is, lasts about ninety seconds before chemically flushing out—if, that is, the person doesn't actively sustain it by trying to avoid it (Taylor, 2006). Of course, a new response may be triggered by a repeated or new thought. But we can easily become trapped in emotional spirals by consciously activating new emotions. If, for instance, you experience a sensation of sadness (which would reach its peak in ninety seconds if you welcome and accept it), it might trigger other thoughts, like "Everyone else is happier than me; my life is worthless." If you buy into such thoughts or get stuck in a broody rut over them, all you're doing is feeding the fire and sustaining your negative feelings.

We also need to convey that emotions aren't always helpful nor do they always carry an important message. Sometimes a past event has conditioned us to react in a certain way, with certain emotions, which in turn triggers thoughts that may not be helpful. This is common if you have experienced a traumatic event, had anxiety in a certain situation, or have a particular phobia. Say that you experience a panic attack at the gym, out of the blue. Later, when you want to return to the gym, your heart starts to race and fear comes up, so you decide not to go to the gym anymore. This is not very helpful in the long run if you value exercising with gym equipment. In this situation, the feeling is not really helpful or guiding you in the right direction. So feelings are not always a great messenger, but it's a better idea to take a look at them than to turn away from them. When you experience emotions, the best thing to do is open up to them, take note of what they are, and leave them be. Forcing emotions, trying to hold on to them or avoiding them, is rarely a fruitful strategy; it leads to a struggle that only makes matters worse.

What the Emotion Is Trying to Tell Me

Understanding our emotions is a key to handling stress more effectively. Here is a quick guide to the messages that basic and universal emotions can convey to us.

Grief. Grief helps us take time to process loss and change and signals to others that we need support and empathy. It can help us activate social networks and can bring together people with similar experiences. Sadness for those we've lost can also help us better appreciate our relationships.

Anger. Anger focuses us on seeking protection, having our way, solving conflicts, righting wrongs, and removing threats. Anger can trigger the fight-or-flight response and release extra energy so we can face a danger or achieve a goal.

Fear. Fear signals that something is wrong or is threatening us. Fear makes us alert and focused on finding out what's wrong. It can help us flee or avoid danger.

Shame. Shame warns us and prevents us from behavior that is possibly disturbing, offensive, or punishable within the prevailing culture and norms.

Guilt. Guilt tells us that we've done something we regret; it can motivate us to put things right while preventing us from making the same mistake again.

Sadness. We get sad when we can't attain important goals in life, when something is taken from us, or when something prevents us from getting or achieving what we want. Sadness can motivate us to make changes in life and set up goals that can take us along the life path we want to travel.

Disgust. Disgust helps us remove ourselves from potentially hazardous situations involving blood, germs, foul-smelling objects that could present a danger, and so on.

Loathing. Loathing is a signal to remove ourselves from something that we dislike, disagree with, or despise, or that can harm us or others.

Interest/curiosity. Interest and curiosity orient us toward things that can please or benefit us. It makes us want to find out more and to approach objects, people, or situations, and it can help us cultivate new skills and contacts.

Joy. Joy signals that we like what we're doing or the situation we're in. Joy helps us bond with other people and allows us to relax, take in new knowledge and insights, and see things from fresh perspectives.

EXERCISE: WILLINGNESS TO MEET NATURAL STRESS

What kinds of natural stress do you have in your life that you can try meeting with willingness (for example, distressing emotions, thoughts, relationships, bodily worries, mental issues, financial difficulties)? Try to name some specific situations that trigger this natural stress, and explore how meeting them with willingness might play out.

Situation	How I can practice willingness

Angela's Example

This was interesting, a real eye-opener. I usually get wound up when I get stuck in a traffic jam. I get annoyed, tense, and angry. I'll try accepting my emotions and the fact that here I am, traffic is really slow, but it's okay, there is nothing I can do about this situation right now, so I'll stay put and just breathe.

TAKING ACTION: WHAT YOU CAN DO BEFORE READING THE NEXT CHAPTER

Schedule a day for reading Chapter 6 of this book. About a week from now would be good. Make a note in your calendar or set an alarm on your phone.

We'll now give you some small challenges to take on before turning to the next chapter. You can also look back at how you rated your life in your Life Compass at the beginning of this chapter. Ask yourself if there's anything you want to do more or less of and can schedule, and then continue with the following:

- **Practice willingness for natural stress.** Acknowledge the presence of natural stress. Something annoying will probably happen before you read the next chapter—you might miss the bus, or you may find yourself up against something more serious. The challenge is to see if you can be willing to have the emotions that rise up inside you. If it's something relatively serious, try the "Healing Hand" exercise. We'd like you to stop, take note of what's going on and how you feel, and open up to your emotional reaction instead of fighting it. See if you can tap into your curiosity about what is going on—investigate and see! Do this at least twice before reading the next chapter.

- **Embrace a value.** Make time for one value in an area of your choosing. Take at least one concrete step and complete at least one activity or behavior associated with the value in question. Pick a small step, something easy to do.

- **Recovery.** Schedule at least two restorative activities and do them.

- **Exercise.** Schedule two (or more) pulse-raising exercise sessions (at minimum a brisk thirty-minute walk).

- **Mindfulness.** Schedule at least one mindfulness exercise.

FOLLOW JOHN AND ANGELA IN THEIR EFFORTS TO LIVE A MORE MEANINGFUL AND BALANCED LIFE

Angela

Willingness for natural stress

I'll try making room for the natural stress I feel when I'm stuck in a traffic jam. I'll also try it when I take the bus and it is late and I miss the first morning meetings.

Embrace a value

I've been wanting to read a book for a while, and now I have one I got from Lizzy. I will start reading it on Wednesday evening.

Recovery

This week I thought I'd have a bath at home two evenings. I'll set out a few candles and add essential oil to the water. I'll also ask my partner to pick up a takeout dinner one night.

Exercise

I'll take a walk at lunchtime as before, but make it a little longer. And then I'll take a brisk walk on Thursday evening and on Saturday with my partner.

Mindfulness

I'll do "Body Scanning" on Monday when I get home from work and one of the shorter exercises with my partner on Sunday.

If you want to learn more about acceptance and how to relate to stressful thoughts, the expanded section of this chapter is for you.

CHAPTER 5 EXPANDED SECTION

In this expanded section, we will look more closely at some myths about happiness and present some methods for exploring your own mind. You might find some of the exercises weird or ridiculous—just bear with us and try out our suggestions.

The Myths and Truths of Happiness

Our colleague Dr. Russ Harris describes, in his lectures and books (such as *The Happiness Trap*, 2008, and *The Reality Slap*, 2012), some of the myths and truths surrounding happiness. Here are some examples.

MYTH #1: HAPPINESS IS OUR NATURAL STATE OF BEING

There is a conception in our society that happiness is actually our natural state of being. This can make us reason that "if I can just get rid of my stress I'll finally be happy!" However, our emotional state is actually in constant flux. No emotional state, be it joy or grief, lasts forever. All we can be sure of is that emotional states, like the weather, are forever changing. That's what it means to be human.

MYTH #2: HAPPINESS MEANS HAVING POSITIVE FEELINGS

Our culture often conveys the notion that happiness means having lovely, positive feelings. But given the basic emotions that all humans have, regardless of culture or ethnicity, striving for only positive feelings is clearly a battle against human nature. Of our ten basic emotions, only two fall neatly into a "positive" category: joy and curiosity. The others are fear, shame, grief, anger, guilt, sadness, disgust, and loathing.

MYTH #3: IF YOU'RE NOT HAPPY, YOU'RE A FAILURE

The notion that happiness means enjoying a steady stream of positive moments can make us feel ashamed and guilty if we're not constantly happy, or beat ourselves up for failing to sustain a state of joy or curiosity. A happy life actually encompasses all kinds of emotions, unpleasant as well as pleasant. It's part of what it means to be human—no one in the history of humankind has managed to stay rooted in only positive emotions. Since the advent of social media, we're also in greater danger of comparing ourselves with others and of seeing only their polished, successful exteriors. Successful people, we may well conclude, are immune to distressing thoughts and negative emotions.

The Acceptance Slider Metaphor

Metaphors are frequently used in ACT because they can sometimes help us get a new perspective of how aspects of our lives relate to each other, and hopefully add some wisdom to our daily life. The slider is a metaphor about acceptance. Imagine that we have two invisible controls inside us, like the volume and tone controls from an old '70s stereo (see Figure 5).

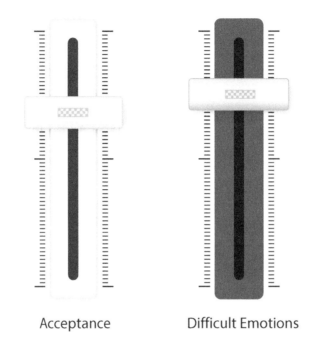

Acceptance   Difficult Emotions

Figure 5: Acceptance slider

The left-hand "acceptance slider" represents our willingness to live with the emotions we have. We have complete control of this slider, and when we accept irritating emotions, it's pushed all the way up to the top. When we're angry with ourselves for feeling stressed or unhappy, the slider is set low— we're not tolerating the fact that our emotions are what they are, and we want to somehow undo what's already been done. But it doesn't matter what we want to do, since we don't have a time machine!

To the right of the acceptance slider is the "difficult-emotions slider." Unfortunately, we have no control over this one; it has a mind of its own.

There is, however, a secret built-in function here, and some people have figured it out. When the acceptance slider is all the way down, when we resist what is already felt, the difficult-emotions slider is always all the way up. It's like it gets stuck there, tormenting us. The unpleasant emotions are at the maximum setting, and no matter how much we try to oil the slider or clear the grit that we think might have jammed it, it refuses to budge. But some people have discovered a secret: when we push the acceptance slider up again, opening up to our emotions no matter how difficult they may feel, it's as if the difficult-emotions slider is released and can move down and up again according to what we are feeling. But as soon as we drag the acceptance slider down again, the difficult-emotions slider goes right to the top and jams again. This is how our thoughts and emotions work, depending on whether or not we accept them. Maybe you've heard the saying "What you resist persists." When we stop resisting and instead create space for difficult emotions, they are free to move, although we have no ultimate control of *how* they move.

How Willingness Can Save You from Drowning

A participant in one of our ACT courses told us how acceptance had saved her from drowning. In the course, we use the quicksand metaphor. It goes like this: Imagine that you've stepped into quicksand. You slowly start to sink, and you panic. Your brain knows only one way to deal with danger: flee. So, with your brain going, "Get out of here!" you lift one foot to try to step back onto solid ground. But all you've done is halve the area over which your weight is distributed. Two feet have become one foot, the pressure increases, and you sink deeper into the sand. Your brain, however, is sticking to the same strategy: "Get out of here!" So you lift your sinking foot and push down with the other one to try to free yourself. But you just sink even deeper. You tread and tread and try to escape, but you just descend deeper and deeper into the muck.

This is a metaphor for how we sometimes struggle with ourselves, with our own emotions. We do everything we can to flee them, but the more we try to break free—as we might do during a panic or anxiety attack—the worse they get. The secret—the tactic that helps you extract yourself from quicksand in real life—is to do the exact opposite of what your brain is telling you to do and create as much surface contact with the sand as you can. When you lie down on your back, you distribute your body weight over a larger area and you can float, a position from which you can call for help or slowly roll away out of danger. Research shows that the same principle also applies to emotions and thoughts (e.g., Gil-Luciano, Ruiz, Valdivia-Salas, & Suárez, 2016; Gillanders, Sinclair, MacLean, & Jardine, 2015). When we fight them, they just get stronger and we become more obsessed with what we're trying to avoid. This is called "ironic processing."

A participant in an ACT workshop told us that once, when she was swimming in the ocean, she found herself in a dense mass of floating seaweed. As she started to struggle she was being dragged deeper into the water. She then followed the standard advice for quicksand: she stopped struggling and leaned back so her weight was distributed over the carpet of seaweed. She was then able to call for help. Her presence of mind possibly saved her life. When we find ourselves engulfed by emotional seaweed, we can remind ourselves that our feelings are natural and harmless. We can practice letting them be—we can lie back and float. It might not be pleasant, but we won't be making it any worse.

Treating Thoughts as Thoughts

What's going on in your mind is just that: something going on in your mind; it is not reality in itself. The fact that you think something doesn't mean it is true, even though you may often feel it is. The exercises we present here use the process of cognitive defusion to create a healthy distance from what's going on in your mind—in other words, treating thoughts as what they are, thoughts, no more, no less. And there is good scientific evidence that such exercises actually do work (e.g., A-Tjak et al., 2015; Levin, Hildebrandt, Lillis, & Hayes, 2012; Healy et al., 2008).

One faculty that sets us apart from other animals is that of language. Language is a blessing in many, many ways—we can plan and create new things, engage in symbolic reasoning, and, above all, communicate with and understand each other. But there is a downside. Language also, for instance, allows us to constantly judge ourselves and label ourselves with words like "useless," "worthless," or "hopeless." In the real physical world, that world we experience through our five senses, "worthless" doesn't exist. It's not an intrinsic property of anything, let alone ourselves. It's just a word, and a word is nothing but a particular combination of sounds, and sounds are just vibrations in our heads caused by airwaves. This might sound strange. We're so used to thinking in words and images that we overlook the fact that thoughts don't actually exist in the material world outside ourselves. Let's do a little experiment. Close your eyes and imagine very vividly a lemon, a really yellow, sour lemon. Imagine taking a bite of this lemon and notice what happens in your mouth. Notice the fresh smell of the lemon. Maybe you're picturing where the lemon was grown or how you'd like to use it to make a tasty drink. Make your image of the lemon as realistic and vivid as possible.

Now we'd like you to, for real, pick up this lemon and cut it in half.

But where did it go? Does this lemon you just thought of exist in reality? Or is it just in your mind? Sure, it's funny that it seems self-evident that the lemon was merely a thought; there's nothing in the world that would convince us otherwise. But when it comes to harsh judgments and thoughts about ourselves—like that we're not good enough, or we're phony, selfish, boring, stupid, or ugly—we can convince ourselves that they're real and objectively true. The next time you become snared in self-judgment, ask yourself: "Is this a yellow lemon that's come to call?" This of course also applies to "I am great," " I am so kind," "I am so beautiful"—all these are just words in our minds and not physical truths. You are who you are, beyond any judgment the mind comes up with.

The exercises that follow can help you start to treat thoughts as thoughts, as mere mental chimera. You can practice these any time, especially when thoughts seem to tangle with you and you feel stuck. Creating a healthy distance from your thoughts and creating more flexibility around your feelings takes time; these exercises are not a quick fix or trick. We suggest that you practice them daily if you find yourself getting caught in thoughts in an unhelpful way.

EXERCISE: DISENGAGE MENTALLY

This exercise is a little noisy, so find a place where you won't be disturbed, or disturb others. First, write down a judgmental thought about yourself that you tend to get hung up on:

_____

_____

Now instead of just thinking this sentence to yourself, sing it aloud to the tune of "Happy Birthday to You." Observe now what happens to the sentence when you sing it instead of just think it.

We also suggest that you listen to a related exercise, "The Chattering Monkey," which you can download as an audio file from http://www.newharbinger.com/41283.

What did you experience when singing the thought for a while? What happened to the thought and the feelings?

_____

_____

EXERCISE: CHANGE THE TYPEFACE OF YOUR THOUGHTS

For this exercise, again write down a judgmental thought you have about yourself. You can use the same one you used previously if you like.

_____

_____

Shut your eyes and do your best to see the thought written down as if on a screen. Now use your mind's eye to adjust the font and typeface of this text. Make the letters huge or tiny. Use bold and italics, only uppercase or only lower. You get the drift. Do this for a few minutes and notice what happens to the thought when you see it like this instead of just thinking it. If you'd like, you could also actually do this exercise on a computer: write down your sentence and change the typeface and size multiple times.

What did you experience when playing with your thoughts this way? What happened to the thought and the feelings?

_____

_____

EXERCISE: WHO AM I?

This exercise can bring some perspective to your cognitive processes and how you use language. It can also help you connect with what we call the "observing self." When you're in touch with this part of yourself, it's often easier to accept thoughts and emotions and not identify yourself so closely with what the thoughts are telling you. The observing self is what we term that part of you that has always observed and experienced everything. Ever since childhood, you've had a perspective from which you've viewed the world—the observing self. Emotions, thoughts, and sensations are always changing, but the observing self is stable and constant. You don't have to try to understand this theoretically; just do your best to stay open to the exercise.

Set a timer for three minutes and make sure you are not disturbed. For three minutes, try to answer the following question (it can be helpful to close your eyes during the exercise). *If you're not allowed to use words or images to describe who you are, who are you?*

There is, of course, no answer to this question, as you can't use words. You must go beyond language, and maybe you realize how language can limit the definition of who you are. At the same time, you're still here; you are still here experiencing yourself and the world; nothing has changed.

The Observing Self

An exercise called "The Observing Self" is another means of connecting with that constant, immutable part of yourself. You can listen to an audio version at http://www.newharbinger.com/41283. We recommend that you listen to it somewhere where you won't be disturbed. The exercise runs for twelve minutes.

How to Handle The Chattering Monkey

In the introduction to this book we described an imaginary chattering monkey on your shoulder, constantly criticizing you. We also mentioned that ACT is about changing your approach to that monkey. This chapter has been about just that. Life will be painful and stressful, and how you approach those experiences determines whether you add unnecessary stress and pain or not. How you approach your thoughts—as "truths" or as what they really are: just thoughts, no more, no less—will also affect your level of unnecessary stress. The next chapter will give you tools to navigate through when life brings on storms.

Willingness: For the Advanced Avoider

Pain in this life is not avoidable, but the pain we create avoiding pain is avoidable.

—R. D. Laing

The most important thing in life that is never addressed in our formal education is how to navigate our inner landscape. We study language, math, physics, geography, and history, but what about relationships, being a good friend, being a parent, or simply dealing with being human? To put it bluntly, our culture offers us two ways of dealing with difficult things in life: to avoid them, or to grit our teeth and carry on. The problem is, these approaches typically generate more stress. Thankfully, there are alternative and much better ways to deal with the storms of life, and that's what this chapter is about. But first, a check-in.

SO HOW ARE YOU DOING?

We predicted that something difficult, either trivial or serious, would probably happen in your life before you read this chapter. Not because you're unlucky, but because difficult things are part of life—they happen all the time. We asked you to stop and acknowledge any challenging feelings and thoughts that surfaced when these difficult experiences occurred, and to possibly try the "Healing Hand" exercise. How did it go?

Completed?	Yes	Partly	No
Practiced willingness for natural stress (acknowledged and willingly opened up to challenging feelings and thoughts)	Yes	Partly	No

On a scale of 0 to 10, how welcoming and accepting were you to your challenging thoughts and feelings?

0 ———————————— 5 ———————————— 10

Not at all welcoming   Very welcoming

If you actively stopped, acknowledged, and opened up to your challenging feelings and thoughts, how did that feel? Was there any difference in how that felt, as opposed to how you have felt when you haven't taken such an accepting approach to your unwanted thoughts and feelings? Write down any differences that you noted:

_____

_____

_____

_____

_____

_____

Now let's follow up on how your other activities went.

Answer these questions and rate how restorative each activity was on a scale of 0 (no recovery) to 10 (plenty of recovery).

Activity	Completed?			Recovery, 0 to 10?
Embraced a value	Yes	Partly	No	
Did at least two recovery activities	Yes	Partly	No	
Exercised at least twice	Yes	Partly	No	
Practiced mindfulness at least once	Yes	Partly	No	

External Events That Got in the Way

If you replied "No" to any of these questions, please note any external events that got in the way of your completing the activity. How could you overcome these obstacles in the future?

Activity	External obstacle	Ideas on how I can deal with this
Embraced a value		
Did two recovery activities		
Exercise		
Mindfulness		

Internal Responses That Showed Up

Write down any challenging thoughts, emotions, or physical sensations that showed up, and how willingly you approached them, when doing your workouts and mindfulness sessions, taking short breaks, or trying new sleeping habits.

Activity	Internal responses (feelings, thoughts, bodily sensations)	On a scale from 0 to 10, how willing was I to experience these feelings, emotions, or sensations?
Embraced a value		
Did two recovery activities		
Exercise		
Mindfulness		

How Have You Been Embracing Your Values?

It's again time to assess your ratings on your Life Compass. How many steps have you taken this past week in the different areas? Remember, your score is completely subjective and based solely on your own personal circumstances, limitations, and goals. Indicate a score for each area and factor in all of the actions you've identified as important, in each area, bearing in mind both quantity and quality.

What does your Life Compass loop for the past week look like?

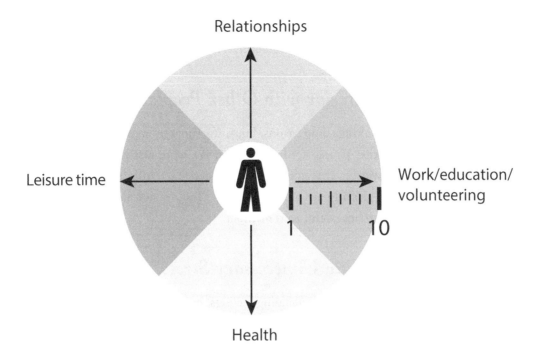

With your Life Compass ratings in mind, is there anything you'd want to do more or less of over the coming week? Some area you'd like to give more priority to? It's best to choose small, attainable goal-related actions.

_____

_____

_____

_____

KEY POINTS FROM CHAPTER 5

Life Hurts Sometimes

We can be easily tempted to value and embrace only those days in life when things are going well and everything feels good. When the going gets tough and life's an uphill struggle, we think we've failed, and we might forget that we don't have total control over life. We might blame ourselves when we're feeling down or unhappy at work or any other area of our life. We are adding this hurtful blame on top of the natural unhappiness or pain that sometimes is a part of life. What good does that do us?

We Compare Our Interior with Other People's Exteriors

Our brains are experts at making comparisons, but unfortunately we fail to see the whole picture. It may seem to us as if most other people are better off, as if they're just happily sailing through life. Again, social media often reinforces this conviction. But everyone suffers, everyone has their own personal struggles and doubts—it's all part of being human. You are not alone in struggling; you're in good company, and sometimes that's useful to remember.

Willingness Can Reduce Unnecessary Stress

When we experience stress or other challenging feelings, we tend to resist, ignore, or try to change them. We judge them and tell ourselves, "I'm a failure" or "It shouldn't be like this." But these judgments just exacerbate our pain. By developing the ability to meet life's challenges, stress, and pain with an open, nonjudgmental mind, we can stop going to war with ourselves and adding unnecessary pain. Being a whole person means experiencing the entire range of emotions—including the challenging ones.

CORE SECTION: STRATEGIES FOR EXPERT AVOIDERS

Many of us would happily be spared from challenging thoughts and feelings, and at least in our Western culture we have long been under the impression that we can avoid challenging feelings by simply "moving on"—forgetting, ignoring, getting our act together, putting on a brave face, or thinking of something else. Many of us had parents who avoided discussing or showing their emotions, who just shut down or physically left the room. We never got the chance to learn that it's possible to allow, show, and discuss challenging feelings, that emotions aren't shameful, ugly, or bad.

To put it simply, our culture offers us two ways of dealing with difficult things in life: avoid or perform (see Figure 6). *To avoid* means just that: we try to avoid feeling what we're feeling, to shut off our emotions and leave behind situations that cause distress, even though they might be meaningful. *To perform* is about keeping ourselves busy and so preoccupied that we don't notice what we're feeling; it's about doing our best to temporarily silence our inner critic. We can also "perform" to prevent ourselves from losing face or status. Any of these ways of approaching life and difficult events eventually generates more stress. Fortunately, there is a third alternative: to be mindful in the pursuit of our values. We'll spend the next few pages exploring these three categories in more detail.

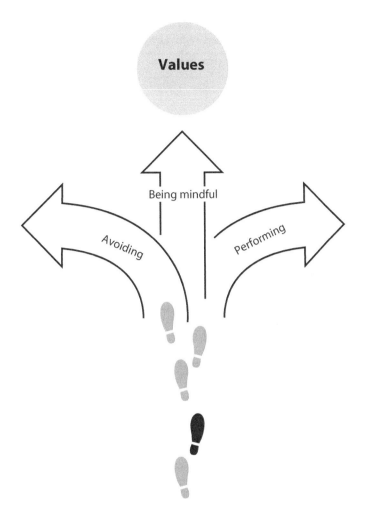

Figure 6: Avoiding, performing, or being mindful

Avoiding

When we're the avoiding version of ourselves, we spend time doing things that spare us from having to feel worry and anxiety, from making fools of ourselves, or from something that feels difficult to do or not do. Maybe we turn down a dinner invitation because we feel insecure, drink alcohol to dampen our emotions, or don't apply for that exciting job to avoid having to be judged in the interview. Or maybe we don't ask for help to avoid seeming incompetent, or we stop seeing a friend who's behaved badly instead of taking the problem up with them. We might say no (or even yes) to something because we fear that to say otherwise could somehow expose a "weakness." Avoidance might bring us away from pain in the short term, but in the long run we may be turning our back on our values. Of course, there are times when saying no could be driven by our values and serve us well—say, when we turn down a dinner invitation because we need recovery time to ourselves—so when we're inclined to avoid, we must always ask ourselves: "Does this bring me toward something I value or away from it?"

Performing

Sometimes we do *more* of things, either to distract ourselves or to try to change what we're feeling. When we use performance as an avoidance technique, we do things mainly to earn ourselves a pat on the back. Maybe we're worried about being exposed as boring, stupid, incompetent, mediocre, a failure, or phony. To be spared these feelings and thoughts, we make sure to do everything twice as well as usual, like work overtime, spend our free time preparing for work, study extra hard, train extra intensively, go on a strict diet, or seek perfection in everything we do. Or we might be overly friendly or concerned about other people's well-being, say yes to every request despite an already packed calendar, or obsessively clean our homes so as not to feel bad when we have visitors. If we perform to avoid the discomfort and pain that naturally accompany life, it can often bring relief, but only temporarily, as the feeling of being competent and good lasts for only so long; there is always something else waiting to be done well. In the long run, this approach usually just creates more stress and increases the risk of fatigue or burnout. At this point, it is easy to lose sight of what we value, and we may give up something we value (such as a job, a partner, or a hobby) because we are burned out, not because we don't still value it. The avoiding and performing categories of human behavior are very similar, and it can be hard to determine which one is dominant in any given situation. But worrying about correct categorization misses the point; the three categories merely offer a tool to help you discover and explore why and how you do the things you do. They help you ask yourself why you are doing what you are doing: whether you are moving *toward* what you value or *away* from what is scary but meaningful to you. Ultimately, this is one of the most important questions you can ask yourself.

Being Mindful: Willingness to Stand the Heat and Act Wisely

When you're the mindful version of yourself, you don't generate that much unnecessary stress, and you act in ways that can help you move toward what is meaningful to you. You acknowledge the difficulties you're experiencing and are more willing to stay open to the emotions they elicit in you. You also make note of the thoughts passing through your mind without letting them steer you away from your life values. When you're being mindful, you do things mainly because they correspond to what is personally significant. You're also more mentally present in what you're doing, unlike when the avoider or the performer in you is calling the shots. You're driven by a desire *toward* or *to* something you consider important: "I clean my home because I value tidiness and beauty, I invite my friends to dinner because I like being with them, and I accept a job because it looks exciting."

The good news is that you can choose to change why you are doing something whenever you like. If you find yourself frantically cleaning as the performer, you can decide to do something else. Being the mindful version of yourself, you can accept what you're actually feeling and keep on tidying up, but for a new reason. Maybe you simply like an ordered house. Or you decide, being mindful, to try something new, like ditching your cleaning project and grabbing a book to read, surrounded by clutter. You'll probably want to start cleaning up eventually. But hopefully then you'll be doing it more mindfully, on the basis of a free, deliberate choice that is consistent with a value, and not compulsively as the performer.

Next, you'll identify behaviors that you think express *avoidance* and *performance* in different situations in your life. No behavior is always avoiding or performing per se; what's important is the *reason* why you are doing it. So *you* need to ascertain whether you're engaged in avoiding or performing behavior, and when you are mindfully moving toward a meaningful activity. Read Angela's example, then write down your own long- and short-term consequences of acting in an avoiding or performing way. Are your actions helpful or unhelpful in the long run? And are they consistent or inconsistent with your values?

Example: Angela's Performance Behaviors

Situation	Performance behaviors	Consequence, short-term	Consequence, long-term
At work, when new tasks are being allocated	I say yes before anyone else.	I feel competent and supporting of the team.	I take on too many jobs and get overworked.
At home, when we're having guests visit	I have to bake my own bread and have the kitchen tidied before they arrive.	I feel pleased to be able to offer them something wholesome. I'm stressed and irritable while baking and cleaning, and I take it out on my partner.	I don't take care of myself and deviate from my life value of not getting entangled in worries and shoulds. To top things off, my partner gets fed up with me, and it sours the evening.

Tip: If you're having difficulty identifying your performing or avoiding behaviors, ask your partner or a good friend. They'll certainly be able to help you!

Your Performance Behaviors

Situation	Performance behaviors	Consequence, short-term	Consequence, long-term

Your Avoidance Behaviors

Situation	Performance behaviors	Consequence, short-term	Consequence, long-term

Now we would like you to challenge the performer and avoider roles and let the mindful version of you take over.

Given your current situation, are there any performance or avoidance behaviors that you'd like to challenge so that you can become more mindful and pursue your values?

Avoidance or performance behaviors: _____

_____

_____

_____

What values, if any, are your avoidance and performance actions related to?

_____

_____

_____

_____

If you were to be mindful and open to the challenging thoughts and feelings (without buying into them) and act more in line with your values, what could you actually *do* instead?

_____

_____

_____

_____

What thoughts and feelings might surface that you would need to make room for (without buying into them)?

_____

_____

_____

_____

John's Example

Avoidance behaviors: *I don't ask for help at work when I feel I'm getting nowhere with a customer.*

Related value: *To be open and vulnerable, to seek contact.*

Do differently: *Try asking for help the next time I get stuck.*

Open to feelings/thoughts: *Feelings of incompetence, fear, doubt; worrying thoughts that people will think I'm a poor team leader.*

Next, we'll guide you through a more advanced willingness exercise.

EXERCISE: WILLINGNESS STANCE

This exercise can help you be mindful when facing challenging thoughts and feelings. You can either read the exercise here or be guided by the audio file that you can stream or download from http://www.newharbinger.com/41283.

1. Take a comfortable seat and, if you like, close your eyes. Become aware of your breathing—your natural, calm, steady breathing that you do without trying to influence it. Take a minute or two and explore your breathing further with these questions:

    Are your breaths deep or shallow?

    Is your breathing rhythm slow or fast?

    Where in your body do you feel yourself breathing?

2. Bring to mind an irritating, stressful thought about yourself, someone else, or a situation. Bring it into your body and take note of what happens to your breathing and your body. Remember,

you don't have to judge or think anything about this experience; just register what happens. After a minute or so, let the thought go and consciously return to your natural, calm breathing. Stay with this natural breathing for a minute.

3. With a curious and open attitude, once again bring that stressful thought to mind and see if you can welcome it into your calm and natural breathing. Consciously give room and allowance for the thought and feeling to land in your breathing and in your body. Note what happens to this painful thought when it is received in your natural, welcoming, and mindful breathing.

4. After a minute or so, become aware of your whole body and your surroundings and emerge from the completed exercise.

What are your reflections from this exercise?

_____

_____

_____

_____

_____

The exercise is one of many ways you can approach your difficult feelings and thoughts without crumbling in the face of life's demands. By breathing into, and opening up to, whatever is there, you make a bit more room for being human and meeting yourself where you are: in the present, a place where you actually live, and which is often more useful and comfortable than living in the past or future. We suggest you bring this exercise into your daily life whenever you meet a challenging situation or feeling; you may even begin to bring a sense of intrigue and curiosity to what is happening inside you, which is often a sign of willingness.

TAKING ACTION: WHAT YOU CAN DO BEFORE READING THE NEXT CHAPTER

Schedule a day for reading Chapter 7 of this book. About a week from now would be good. Make a note on your calendar or set an alarm on your phone.

The Mindfulness & Acceptance Workbook for Stress Reduction

We'll now suggest some activities to do before you move on to the next chapter. Remember not to be too ambitious; better to succeed at something small than fail at something big.

You can also look back at how you rated your life in your Life Compass at the beginning of this chapter. Is there anything you want to do more or less of and can schedule? Then continue with the following:

- **Practice willingness for natural stress.** Something annoying will probably happen before you read the next chapter—you might misplace your keys or find yourself up against something more serious. See if you can make room for the emotions that arise. If it's something relatively serious, try the "Healing Hand" exercise from Chapter 5. Stop, take note of what's going on and how you feel, and open up to your emotional reaction instead of fighting it. See if you can be curious about what is going on. Do this at least twice.

- **Challenge performance or avoidance behaviors.** Take note of what thoughts and feelings come to the surface when you act mindfully, and make room for them. It could be helpful to write down your thoughts and feelings by completing the sentences: "I'm having the thought that …" and "I'm having a feeling of …"

- **Recovery.** Schedule at least two restorative activities, small enough for you to confidently commit to.

- **Exercise.** Schedule two (or more) pulse-raising exercise session (at minimum, a brisk thirty-minute walk).

- **Mindfulness.** Schedule at least one mindfulness exercise and do it.

FOLLOW JOHN AND ANGELA IN THEIR EFFORTS TO LIVE A MORE MEANINGFUL AND BALANCED LIFE

John

Accepting natural stress

This exercise is great now that I've given it a try. I'll continue to accept natural stress when it crops up. For example, I notice that I get stressed about being stressed. But what good does that do? I'll just stop and accept the natural stress I get when I feel short of time, note its existence, and not get worked up over it.

Challenging performance or avoidance behaviors

I'll challenge my performance behavior and stop meticulously preparing my team meetings.

Related values: Working in a balanced way.

Allow and do differently: I'll go through my presentation just once instead of three times.

Accept: I'll get all apprehensive and worried that I'll screw up or forget something. I'll accept these feelings and let them hang around like a radio playing in the background.

Recovery activities

I'll make sure I'm free again on Sunday and go for a bike ride in the woods. I'll take a packed lunch and download a podcast to listen to. I'll have a rest and listen to a podcast on Tuesday after work too. I've also scheduled a nice long lunch with myself on Wednesday.

Exercise

I'll continue cycling to work and am going to try out a CrossFit session in the gym on Wednesday. On Friday I'll do a full session at the gym. I'll keep on doing my hourly stretching at work.

Mindfulness

I'll do the "Breathing Anchor" today after finishing this chapter and again before the team meeting on Tuesday.

Do you find yourself sometimes getting hung up on debilitating thoughts? Do you want some tips about how to get over life's hurdles? If so, the expanded section of this chapter might be of help.

CHAPTER 6 EXPANDED SECTION

When you take a step toward what you consider important in life, insecurity and other challenging thoughts and feelings will be joining you. These thoughts and feelings often serve to protect us—they are part of our wonderful brain, which is programmed to predict all problems and steer us away from potential disaster. But sometimes we let our thoughts, feelings, and memories obstruct us from doing what we want. So we'll be focusing now on how you can negotiate these obstacles, on both the outside and the inside.

External and Internal Obstacles

We're often able to change and influence things that happen in the external world by adopting strategies like problem solving. At other times, it's worth accepting that some things are difficult or take time to change. When it comes to internal obstacles and hurdles—by which we mean our own thoughts and feelings—it's often healthy to accept their presence in the here and now. This does not mean that they are in any way true. It's hard to control our thoughts, and even the most successful people have dark thoughts and feelings about themselves. We've been duped into believing that we need self-confidence to follow our own path in life—and that having self-confidence means being free from doubt and insecurity. Research shows, however, that we develop our self-confidence by doing, and doing well, things that we haven't dared to do before (e.g., Baumeister, Campbell, Krueger, & Vohs, 2003). What's paramount is the *action*, not the thought. By taking on challenges, we learn—we grow and become better at listening to our needs and following our values. Let's look at how we can approach our inner obstacles and challenges wisely.

HANDLING OUR INNER OBSTACLES

Surprisingly, many obstacles we encounter in life come from within. We have thoughts like "I can't," "It would never work," "I don't dare." Now imagine the following scenario, no matter how irrelevant it seems to your life:

You're single and interested in a colleague you've seen a few times in your company's large dining room. You want to ask this person to have a coffee with you—maybe as a step toward starting a relationship. But you're incredibly nervous about being turned down. You're standing in the dining room, and this person is standing just a few feet away, and you're just about to make your approach. But at that moment, a whole load of thoughts enters your head, making it hard for you to make your move. These thoughts want only what's best for you; they just want to shield you from any emotional pain your daring move might cause. Maybe you have memories of making a fool of yourself in the past, or maybe you've been let down by someone. Whatever it is, your thoughts and feelings want to protect you from a repeat experience.

Thoughts that pop into your head are:

"He or she will say no."

"I'll just be making a fool of myself."

"I'm not attractive enough."

"I lack the self-confidence."

When these or similar thoughts arise, you can approach them in different ways:

1. **Listen to the thoughts, buy them, and adapt.** Maybe you normally feel you should heed the thoughts because they have something important to say, and maybe you remember how you were let down in the past. In the situation just described, this would mean that, believing the thoughts to be true, you adapt to them by different means, for example:

   - Rehearsing replies to all the possible things the person might say so as not to make a fool of yourself

   - Buying new clothes that seem more matched to the person's style before you make your move

   - Putting it off for another day, because you're nervous and don't want to be caught blushing

   - Buying a book on how to boost your self-confidence instead of approaching the person right away

   Strategies like these take a lot of energy and often remove your focus from what you actually want. They're rarely that effective, and the chances of getting an affirmative response—and of moving in the direction in which you want to go—are no greater. On the contrary, your adaptive strategy prevents you from acting, and you've started to direct your attention and energy toward being perfect and minimizing risks.

2. **Boost your self-confidence.** A common strategy is trying to boost one's self-confidence by trying to change one's feelings and thoughts. We try to overcome the negative thoughts using positive ones, arguments, or what are known as "affirmations": "I'm great, and I know it"; "I've got a nice body, I love my body"; "Many of my friends say I'm good-looking"; "I'm actually pretty smart." We call this "cognitive karate," and the problem is, the thoughts we're trying to silence tend to shout even louder. It takes a lot of energy to continually keep negative thoughts at bay and to think positively. It's likely the strategy will bring you no closer to making that date with the intriguing coworker, and this internal karate fight may just recall previous failures.

3. **Be mindful of the thoughts and feelings—and act.** A more sustainable strategy is to be mindful of these thoughts, accepting that they appear and that they are a part of being a human being. In practice, this entails letting the thoughts exist and going ahead with your mission regardless. Your being turned down or not isn't the point; what matters is that you've taken a step toward something you value, and that is the only thing you actually can control: your steps. Unfortunately, your accelerating pulse and the thoughts that still torment you are beyond your direct influence, as is the other person's answer. But by approaching and talking to the object of your desire, instead of attending a self-confidence course, you've greatly improved your chances of a date. In other words, it's better to put energy into what you *can* change—and not what you *can't*. As hockey star Wayne Gretzky once said: "You miss scoring a goal in 100 percent of the shots you don't take."

EXERCISE: MEETING YOUR INNER OBSTACLES AND CHALLENGES

We'll now take you through six steps for dealing with the obstacles on your way toward something important. Think about your Life Compass; is there a step that you feel you want to take in your life right now? An area in which you don't feel secure, that can elicit feelings of doubt and negative thoughts? Write it down here.

1. An important step I want to take

_____

_____

_____

_____

John's Example

An important step: *I'd like to start singing in a chorus.*

2. Obstacles

If you think about taking this step, what inner obstacles in the form of thoughts and feelings do you get that can make it hard for you? Write them down here. In this situation you don't have to judge how "true" a thought/obstacle is. Just make a note of the thoughts that come into your mind.

I'm having the thought that … _____

I'm having the thought that … _____

I'm having the thought that … _____

I'm having a feeling of … _____

I'm having a feeling of … _____

I'm having a feeling of … _____

John's Example

I'm having the thought that *I can't sing.*

I'm having the thought that *once the other kids laughed at me when I sang in school.*

I'm having the thought that *if there's an audition I'll fail it.*

I'm having a feeling of *fear.*

I'm having a feeling of *being sick to my stomach.*

Next, let's look at impulses—those seemingly irresistible responses you are subject to when you have these uncomfortable thoughts and feelings.

3.   Impulses

_____

_____

_____

_____

John's Example

Impulses: *Don't bother to check out the choruses in town; put off a decision until later; take private singing lessons instead of joining a chorus.*

4. Can you make room for your thoughts and feelings?

We'll now ask you some questions to get you thinking about whether it's really true that these thoughts are obstructing you and that you have to get rid of them.

If we ask ourselves how long we've had these kinds of obstructive thoughts and feelings—when they came into our head for the first time—most of us would say they've been there for ages.

How long have these thoughts and feelings existed for *you*? When was the first time you thought or felt them? Write down an age or the number of years next to your earlier notes.

Do you feel you have to get rid of your thoughts and feelings before taking a step toward your goal?

What are the chances that you'll be able to get rid of them for good?

Have you had negative thoughts and feelings for a long time and in many different contexts and yet still managed to take some steps toward your goal?

The likelihood of your ever being completely rid of these thoughts and feelings is probably close to zero. When we do trivial things, thoughts and feelings like these often lie low. But when we take a step toward something really important in our life, they emerge, because they really want to protect us from pain and distress. Because if something's important to us, there's also a chance that it will hurt us in some way. We'd like to challenge you to practice welcoming and accepting these thoughts and feelings instead:

Welcome these thoughts and feelings, register their existence, and thank them for trying to help you.

You don't have to believe what the thoughts are telling you, and you don't need to disprove them either. Let the thoughts babble on without your wasting energy on them. Try imagining that you've tuned in to some noisy radio station, and let the radio chatter away in the background.

We'll now guide you in an acceptance practice called the "Physicalization Exercise," which can help you coexist mindfully with your negative thoughts and feelings. You can either read it here or be guided by the audio file at http://www.newharbinger.com/41283.

5. The Physicalization Exercise

1. Be seated comfortably and, if you like, shut your eyes. Become aware of your breathing—your natural, calm breathing that you do when not trying to influence it.

    What rhythm does it have?

    Where in your body do you feel yourself breathing?

2. Now think of the negative thoughts and feelings that come into your head when you want to take a step toward something that's important to you. Welcome these, and take note of what

happens to your breathing and inside your body. See if you can get closer to the feeling by listening to what is happening in your body.

3.   Now think of the following questions, one at a time:

Where do you physically feel the feelings in your body? If you want, you can trace a finger around the area of your body the feeling seems to occupy.

If the feeling had a color, what color would it be?

If the feeling had form, what would it be like (hard, cold, sticky, warm, round, glossy)?

If the feeling had mass, how heavy would it be?

Now see if you can breathe into the feeling to supply the area with oxygen. Can you make room for the feeling in your body? Try relaxing your shoulders and hips and breathing deeply, letting your abdomen expand.

When you've breathed with the feeling for a while, you can release your active grip on your mindful breathing and return to the room you're sitting in. Open your eyes and stretch. The exercise is now over.

6.   Act according to your values

You've now gone through an important step in developing the skill of willingness by addressing your impulse to avoid the pain and using acceptance and willingness as a way to meet it. How would you act in accordance with what's important to you instead of obeying your impulses?

_____

_____

_____

_____

Plan and schedule when you want to act on your values with this new perspective.

John's Example

I'll search on the net this evening for a chorus and ask Anders if he knows of any. I'll let my doubts and fears stay where they are, accept them, register that they're there, and thank my brain for trying to stop me from taking unnecessary risks.

Getting Over Life's Hurdles

This chapter has covered helpful strategies to deal with the tough situations you encounter in your life—those that really play on your desire to avoid them. We also showed you how to use certain willingness techniques to confront this avoidance, and so reduce your stress and live the life you desire. In the next chapter, we will discuss relationships—something that most every human needs in order to be content, and a source of vitality for many people (and a source of stress when they are not working). We'll show you how to use willingness to cultivate vital relationships.

Healthy Relationships

Intimacy is the capacity to be rather weird with someone—and finding that's okay with them.

—Alain de Botton

Are you rather strange? Do you think differently and seem to constantly elicit quizzical stares from your friends, including your partner? Is this because you are just being you? Thankfully, we are all different; no two of us are alike. But in a world that expects certain people to act in certain ways, it is a brave person who does not follow that well-trodden path. Whether your meaningful life is traditional and "appropriate," or it is rather eccentric and derives vitality through actions others do not take, being the person you are is the key to healthy and loving relationships—relationships such as those that you, strange as you are, may have with the people who look at you not only quizzically but with deep affection.

Stressful periods in our work and other areas of practical responsibility can sometimes feel very lonely, since relationships tend to slip down on our list of priorities. But few aspects of life are as important for stressed-out people as healthy relationships. As we've indicated, a healthy relationship is one in which you are free to act and communicate your ideas and values: those parts of you that you think others may find strange. However, taking the courage to live in a way that is vital to you tends to communicate a joy and enthusiasm that attracts people with whom you can build healthy relationships. This, of course, requires the courage to take rejection of not only a potential relationship but also what you stand for, which you may perceive as a rejection of *you*. However, to build the healthy relationships that sustain you in stressful times and bring you joy in less-stressful times, you need to be willing to accept your difficult fears and worries and still communicate with some others the actions and interests that make you the person you are.

In previous chapters, we have discussed how you can use willingness to move through such worries and difficult thoughts. In this chapter, we focus on general relationship skills that most people need, whether they are a leader of a nation or a nurse. The foundation of such skills is that of effective communication, so let's look at that.

As usual, we first start out with a check-in and a look back at the key points from the last chapter.

SO HOW ARE YOU DOING?

We predicted that some adverse event, either trivial or serious, would happen before you read this chapter. We asked you to stop and acknowledge any challenging feelings and thoughts that surfaced. How did that go?

Completed?	Yes	Partly	No

On a scale of 0 to 10, how welcoming and accepting were you to your challenging thoughts and feelings?

0 ———————————— 5 ———————————— 10

Not at all welcoming   Very welcoming

If you actively stopped, acknowledged, and accepted your challenging feelings and thoughts from the event, did that approach change how you experienced the event? If so, how?

_____

_____

_____

_____

Did You Manage to Challenge a Performance or an Avoidance Behavior?

You were asked to be mindful and open instead of performing and avoiding on at least one occasion last week. How did it go?

How did you approach any difficult thoughts or feelings that came up?

_____

_____

How Did You Do on Your Other Activities?

Answer these questions and rate how restorative each activity was on a scale of 0 (no recovery) to 10 (plenty of recovery).

Activity	Completed?			Recovery, 0 to 10?
Did at least two recovery activities	Yes	Partly	No	
Exercised at least twice	Yes	Partly	No	
Practiced mindfulness at least once	Yes	Partly	No	

External Events That Got in the Way

If you replied "No" to any of these questions, please note any external events that got in the way of your completing the activity. How could you overcome these obstacles in the future?

Activity	External obstacle	Ideas on how I can deal with this
Did at least two recovery activities		
Exercised at least twice		
Practiced mindfulness at least once		

Internal Responses That Showed Up

Write down any challenging thoughts, emotions, or physical sensations that showed up, and how willing you were to them, when doing your recharging activities physical exercise , t or practicing mindfulness.

Activity	Internal responses (feelings, thoughts, bodily sensations)	Rate how open and allowing you were able to be (1 to 10)
Did at least two recovery activities		
Exercised at least twice		
Practiced mindfulness at least once		

How Have You Been Embracing Your Values?

How much progress have you made this past week in the four areas of values? Remember, your score is completely subjective and based solely on your own personal circumstances. Indicate a score for each area, including all the actions that you've identified as important in each one, bearing in mind both quantity (such as how many times you took an action or how much courage an action took for you) and the quality of how you experienced an action (such as willingly or just putting up with it).

What does your Life Compass look like for the past week?

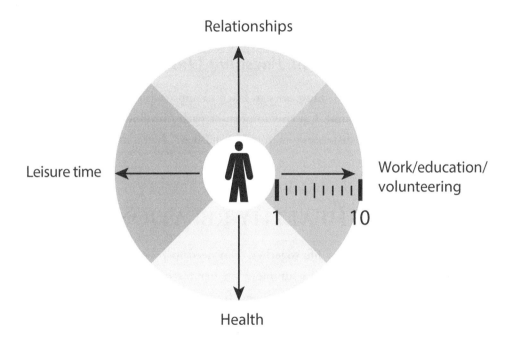

As always, don't worry if it's uneven; different valued areas demand our attention from week to week. But if the imbalance persists you might want to see if you can spend even a little time attending to a neglected value in your life. With your Life Compass rating in mind, is there anything you'd want to do more or less of over the coming week? Some area you'd like to give more priority to? It's best to be realistic in what you choose to do; remember, it's better to do something small than nothing at all.

_____

_____

_____

_____

KEY POINTS FROM CHAPTER 6

We All Want to Avoid Challenging Emotions.

Few of us either are properly trained in meeting challenging emotions or have the luxury of people around us who are experts at listening. We're told that we have to pull ourselves together, to stop crying, to just get on with our lives. Fear of expressing ourselves can make us want to avoid difficult emotions, but when we do, over time our lives become narrower and less fulfilled, not to mention that we are less able to relax or embrace activities, situations, or people that we fear could arouse negative feelings.

Mindfulness Is an Aid in Pursuing Our Values.

Instead of avoiding and performing, we can learn to approach our challenging thoughts and feelings with an open heart and mind. On this important path of following our heart's will we are particularly susceptible to doubt, distressing memories, and fears. Here, mindfulness and compassion are our staunch allies.

CORE SECTION: HEALTHY RELATIONSHIPS

You're just managing to hold your life together. You need to pick up the kids, the company budget needs sorting out, you forgot to call your mom on her birthday, and if that weren't enough, your furnace isn't functioning. How on earth will you find time to keep old friendships alive when you hardly have time for a cup of tea with your partner?

When life is stressful it's easy to let relationships go. But relationships matter. Humans are social animals, and our relationships are important—even vital—to us as a species, never mind as individuals. In one classic study, researchers found that social isolation was even more life-threatening than smoking. With sound relationships, our chances of living longer are 50 percent higher than they are with poor relationships (Holt-Lunstad, Smith, & Layton, 2010; House, Landis, & Umberson, 1988).

Even at work, social relationships are crucial. In fact, good relationships at work, and in general, not only decrease our perceived levels of stress, but also have been shown to affect our genome and strengthen the immune system, so we stay healthier (Cacioppo, Cacioppo, Capitanio, & Cole, 2015; Cole et al., 2015; Davidson & McEwen, 2012; Eisenberger & Cole, 2012; Baruch-Feldman, Brondolo, Ben-Dayan, & Schwartz, 2002).

In this chapter, we'll give you a chance to review your relationships. Maybe you find that some need a little TLC (tender love and caring) and that enhancing your communication skills could strengthen your connection to someone. Since our way of communicating is essential to how our relationships work, we will focus on these important skills.

Communication for Better Relationships

"Aren't you ever coming to bed? You're so … selfish! You don't care that I'm tired."

"Mmm."

"Don't walk off when I'm talking to you!"

"That does it! You're always so pissed off!"

"Me, pissed off? You can talk! You just go around mumbling all the time. I can't talk to you."

Such is the dismal kind of exchange that a tired, irritable couple can have when trying to communicate. Does it sound familiar? It's easy to end up in destructive patterns. Yet there's nothing more important than communication for getting relationships to work. How we communicate—especially on difficult topics or at times when we're tired, angry, or sad—plays a huge part in how happy we are in a relationship, and how healthy we are overall. When we end up in conflict with someone, or want to criticize or give an opinion, there are essentially three ways to communicate: with avoidance, aggressively, or calmly and clearly.

It is, of course, usually most effective to be calm and clear, for reasons that will soon be apparent. We can summarize the characteristics of these three approaches as follows.

AVOIDANCE IN RELATIONSHIPS

Avoidance means choosing not to confront the other person or state what we're thinking or feeling. This approach manifests in many ways, such as:

- Saying nothing

- Withdrawing from the conversation and leaving the room

- Turning attention to something else

- Finding distractions to keep out of the other person's way

- Agreeing (even without saying anything) to avoid conflict

- Making excuses

- Avoiding eye contact

- Turning away from the other person

- Sleeping

- Slouching

- Not finding time to be alone together

- Having sex instead of talking (although sex instead of long, fruitless quarrels can sometimes be beneficial, to bond again)

AGGRESSION

Aggression is another unhelpful communication approach. Being threatening or extremely angry can sometimes be an effective means of gaining compliance from people very quickly—but only in the short term. In the longer term it is very rarely conducive to communication and healthy relationships. Aggressive actions include:

- Rolling your eyes

- Accusing the other person

- Ordering the other person around

- Raising your voice

- Crossing your arms

- Shouting

- Saying nasty things

- Threatening the other person (directly or indirectly)

- Encroaching on the other person's personal space

- Puffing up your chest

- Staring the other person in the eye

- Making the other person do something

- Bullying behaviors, such as not including people in situations or failing to provide them with information they might need in order to fulfill their responsibilities

ACTING WITH CALMNESS AND CLARITY

It's usually most effective to express ourselves in a calm, clear manner. When we do, we improve our chances of being heard and understood, which can help further our own values. This communication approach facilitates conversation and the maintenance of good relationships. When we communicate clearly and calmly, it doesn't necessarily mean that we *feel* calm and clear. But our thoughts and feelings don't need to control our physical actions; even if we are annoyed by someone, we show respect and can get our views and opinions across more effectively if we communicate clearly, calmly, and in a measured tone. We promote mutual understanding and make it easier for ourselves to move the situation toward our valued ends.

Using the calm and clear strategy means, for example:

- Speaking in a normal conversational tone

- Talking descriptively instead of accusingly

- Using "I-messages" (more on these shortly)

- Expressing feelings and thoughts clearly and calmly

- Maintaining relaxed yet steady eye contact

- Turning toward the other person

- Keeping arms and hands relaxed (perhaps by letting them hang naturally)

Let's look more closely at how we can express ourselves with greater calmness and clarity.

Convey a Calm and Clear I-Message

One way of being critical or expressing an opinion that is often very effective is the I-message. This is a fundamental and simple strategy but one that works extremely well. The antithesis of the I-message is the you-message, which comes across as accusatory. A you-message often includes one or more of these elements:

- An accusatory statement about the other person, such as "You're such a …," "You always …" and so forth

- Judgmental, abstract words that ascribe a particular personality trait to the person, such as lazy, boring, irresponsible, sloppy, cruel, or stupid

- The words "never" and "always"

- Reference to former conflicts or wrongs committed by the other person

Here's an example of a you-message:

"You never do the dishes! You don't take responsibility for things! And it's the same with putting away the food. It's always me planning what to buy and cook. Last week I did the shopping every day. You're lazy."

A better alternative is the calm, clear I-message. By using the I-message you can prevent or mitigate conflict. The I-message derives from what *you feel* when someone does a particular action. Expressing an I-message doesn't mean that you always get your way, but it does mean you get to express your experience and desires and what you would like the other person to do differently. I-messages also focus on behavior rather than personality—in other words, you are not ascribing the other person's actions to deep-seated personality problems or a meddlesome mother. It's easier for someone to hear and take in a message about actions he is taking than it is for him to accept criticism of his personality. It's also a better guide for the person: you are pointing out what specific, concrete behavior the person can change.

EXERCISE: USING AN I-MESSAGE TO ENHANCE COMMUNICATION

These are the four fundamental ingredients of an I-message:

1. **The word "I."** The message usually begins with the pronoun "I" (hence the name).

2. **My feeling.** You state your emotional reaction to what the person does, is doing, or has done.

3. **The behavior you want to discuss.** You describe what the other person does or has done that you are reacting to, in the most concrete terms possible.

4. **The consequences of that behavior.** You describe the consequences you fear the behavior will have for your relationship if it continues.

By combining these ingredients, we can produce I-messages of varying levels of complexity. It's best, however, to start at a more basic level and work your way up. For instance:

I + my feeling + the other person's behavior: "I feel irritated when you don't tidy up after yourself."

I + my feeling + the other person's behavior + my desire: "I feel irritated when you don't tidy up after yourself. I'd like to talk about setting up some sort of cleaning schedule."

I + my feeling + the other person's behavior + consequence + my desire: "I feel irritated when you don't tidy up after yourself. It just makes me want to go away and brood. I'd like to talk about setting up some sort of cleaning schedule."

Is there an element in your relationship with someone—a colleague, a friend, a partner, or a relative—that causes irritation and friction and would be good to raise with the person in a calm, clear way? Go through the following section to see if you can formulate your own I-message. Respond to each item in as much detail as possible.

The person's name: _____

Your I-message:

Think of a recurring situation that disturbs or irritates you. What does the person do that elicits these feelings?

_____

_____

_____

_____

How does it make you feel? Describe your emotional response(s).

_____

_____

_____

_____

What consequences do you think this can ultimately have for your relationship if it continues?

_____

_____

_____

_____

What would you prefer the other person do? Suggest things that can increase the chances of you seeing eye-to-eye on this. Focus on the person's behavior.

_____

_____

_____

_____

Now formulate your own I-message on the basis of the preceding criteria. This is only an exercise; it's up to you whether you actually use it or not.

I... _____

_____

_____

_____

Saying Yes and No in Relationships

A fairly common problem for people suffering from troublesome levels of stress is saying yes to too many things to the people around them. They do this for all sorts of reasons: maybe they're overly ambitious or just have difficulty saying no because they are unwilling to experience the stress of doing so. People with stress problems often do tasks by themselves without asking for help. When we say yes to too many things, we risk that those things will become another source of stress, and we limit the actions we can take to live our other values.

Here are some of the common reasons we fail to say no even though saying yes goes against our vital living and instead leads to stress:

- Fear of disappointing other people

- Fear of missing out on something fun or important

- Not knowing what you actually want, so you say yes to whoever seems more insistent or important

- It's nice to say yes; it makes you feel needed, competent, worthy, and important

- Fear of being left out in the future

- Fear of being alone

- Fear of being considered boring

- It sounds fun, and more-of-the-same positive stress won't do you any harm (but of course, it can if it conflicts with more value-motivated activities)

- Other reasons:

  _____

  _____

Keep in mind that when you say no to something, you're also actually saying yes to something else—namely, the opportunity to give yourself something different that you yourself value. Sometimes, of course, you don't know what else you want, but you might know what you don't want to say yes to. In saying no you can give yourself the time and space to explore what you want to say yes to.

There are two mottos that can help you say no effectively:

"I'm not saying no to you but yes to me."

and

"By saying no here, I can keep my yes."

SAYING YES

Being a constant no-sayer is, obviously, not a good long-term strategy—it's inflexible and doesn't allow us to pursue our values. We need to say yes to things we actually want to do! Sometimes we say no to things not because they're unimportant, but because we unquestioningly accept self-assessments like "I won't be able to manage it; that's not for me." Once you become aware of the thoughts and feelings that stop you from saying yes, you can challenge them. Let these difficult thoughts accompany you on your journey when you take the step toward what you consider important in life.

SAYING NO: WHAT YOU CAN DO—IF YOU NEED TO RESPOND, BASED ON YOUR VALUES

We've already looked at how you can communicate calmly, clearly, and firmly with I-messages, and you can also apply the I-message strategy when you need to say no to a request, to be true to your values. Here's some other advice you might find useful:

- Thank the person for asking you for your participation in whatever you are asked about, and then say no. "Oh, that seems fun. Thank you for asking me; I'm glad you thought of me and invited me, and I am sorry I cannot come."

■ If you are not certain if it's a yes or no and need some time to think about it, ask for that time instead of saying yes and perhaps needing to back out later. Many questions don't require an immediate answer, so say you'll get back to them: "Oh, that seems interesting; thank you for asking me. Could you give me some time to think it over? When do you need an answer?"

■ Sometimes we think we have to give a reason other than an outright (or implied) "I don't want to"—a white lie. Many times this can be appropriate, but if you are on good terms with the requester, see if you can try being more honest: "Oh, thanks for asking; that seems interesting, but I'm not really up for it."

■ Consider what you truly want. We often get steamrollered into a yes because we don't know what we want ourselves, so we can easily follow other people's suggestions and take on too much. So take time to consider what you want, especially in situations where you know in advance that you might be asked or might have difficulty refusing.

■ Ask for help in prioritizing or conveying your needs. When someone is asking for your help and you are up to your eyeballs with tasks and commitments, instead of making up an excuse, see if you can explain your situation. If you are interested in participating, ask for help prioritizing.

For example, here's John again, who's up to *his* eyeballs in work and doesn't want to take on any more. What he needs is time for recovery and help with prioritizing his tasks and responsibilities at work. When he's asked to do something, he replies by accompanying his refusal with a vague reason, not really explaining what he actually needs:

John's team leader: "Hi, John! We were wondering if you could take over the new IT project that Kristina's working on, as she's going to be on leave this fall. We'd like you to take over the team meetings that she usually leads on Monday evenings. We think you'd be perfect for the job!"

John: "Er, hmm, I can't on Mondays; that's when I've got my CrossFit sessions."

John's team leader: "Ah … okay … but that's no problem; we can shift the meetings to Wednesday evenings instead."

Using vague reasons, excuses, or white lies can just make things harder for us.

■ It can cause requesters to put on their problem-solver's hat instead of helping you out. In this instance, John's team leader sought to solve John's "problem" by changing the day of the meeting, when in fact John was already maxed out with work, and *if* he were to take on any more tasks he would need help with prioritizing.

- It can cause us to pit one commitment against another, just creating more difficulty. When John gives CrossFit training as his reason, that tells his team leader that John's not sufficiently committed to his role. John could instead point out the inadequate resources of his team and his need for more recovery time.

Think now about activities or suggestions that you automatically say yes to, that are not really in line with your values—or even if they are, you actually need to say no to in order to create more space for yourself right now.

Write them down here along with the value they relate to:

Activity/suggestion to turn down	Related value

What feelings and thoughts would you need to acknowledge when you turn this down?

_____

_____

_____

_____

In an ideal world, what could the long-term benefits be if you managed to say no in these situations?

_____

_____

_____

_____

Angela's Example

I need to say no to having my grandchild's birthday party at my place. I really don't have the energy right now.

Life Value: *Stand up for myself; find balance.*

Acknowledge: *I need to make space for possible feelings of shame and inadequacy. But there's not much I can do about it—I just don't have the energy for a party.*

In an ideal world: *Saying no can help me bring my life more into balance, and I'll be able to say no in other situations in the same way. And the people around me will have more respect for me and my limits.*

Asking for Help

It's quite common for us to not ask for help when we're stressed. We think it's more efficient to perform the task ourselves so we can be sure to get it done promptly and in our preferred way. But in the long run this kind of behavior makes us take on too many tasks that we could actually get help with. According to research (Uchino, 2009; Andre-Petersson, Hedblad, Janzon, & Ostergren, 2006), asking for help not only lightens our workload but also strengthens our relationships. Do you notice that instead of asking for help in a crunch, you almost always try to sort things out yourself? In what areas of your life could you challenge yourself to ask for help? Fill in your responses.

Area	What I could ask for help with	The people I could ask	Related value

When you picture yourself asking for help, what obstacles can you see yourself facing?

_____

_____

_____

_____

How would you handle these obstacles?

_____

_____

_____

_____

Angela's Example

I'd like to ask my son for help now that we're going to redecorate the bedroom. The related life value is to be open and vulnerable and to find balance. I'm not used to asking him for help, as I get the feeling that he'd be annoyed and put-upon. I'm also a little afraid and ashamed that I need help. But I've made up my mind to confront my fear and ask him. I'm willing to experience these challenging feelings and pay little attention to the stories my brain will start telling me. I will keep my focus on how they feel physically.

Note: When you've spent a lifetime taking responsibility and rarely asking for help, the people around you are likely to expect you to continue doing so. When you change your behavior you might meet with resistance at first. Be aware of this, and see if you can take small steps that improve your chances of success.

TAKING ACTION: WHAT YOU CAN DO BEFORE READING THE NEXT CHAPTER

Schedule a day for reading Chapter 8 of this book. About a week from now would be good. Make a note on your calendar or set an alarm on your phone.

Now, here are some activities for you to do before you move on to the next chapter. Remember not to be too ambitious; it's better to succeed at something small than fail at something big. You can also look back at how you rated your life on your Life Compass at the beginning of this chapter. Is there anything you want to do more or less of and can schedule? We suggest that when you take actions related to your Life Compass you find a way of incorporating the following communication strategies, where applicable:

- **Embrace a value.** Make time for one value in an area of your choosing.

- **Change your communication.** Decide to change the way you communicate with someone in your life. Maybe you could use an I-message or say no to someone, or perhaps ask them for help. Schedule when and with whom, and set a reminder to take on this new challenge.

- **Practice willingness for natural stress.** Acknowledge the presence of challenging thoughts and feelings. Something annoying will probably happen before you read the next chapter—you might forget an appointment or find yourself up against something more serious. Your activity is to see if you can open up to the emotions that rise up inside you. If it's something relatively serious, try the "Healing Hand" exercise from the end of Chapter 5 or the "Acceptance" exercise you learned in the previous chapter. In essence, take a deep breath, register what's happening and how you're feeling, and accept your emotional reaction instead of fighting it. Do this at least twice.

- **Recovery.** Schedule at least two recovery activities and do them.

- **Exercise.** Schedule at least two pulse-raising exercise sessions (at minimum, a brisk thirty-minute walk).

- **Mindfulness.** Schedule at least one guided mindfulness exercise from the book's website, http://www.newharbinger.com/41283, and do it.

FOLLOW JOHN AND ANGELA IN THEIR EFFORT TO LIVE A MORE MEANINGFUL AND BALANCED LIFE

Angela

Change in communication

I'll say no to Kristy the next time she asks me to join her and the others for a girls' night out. It's not like we get a lot out of seeing each other, and I really only do it out of a sense of duty. I'll also say no to hosting my grandchild's birthday party, as I just don't have the energy at the moment.

Willingness for natural stress

I'll be open and willing to experience the feelings of shame and inadequacy when I say no to my granddaughter about the party. That's just the way things are at the moment. I just don't have the energy.

Recovery

I'll meet Debbie on Saturday; we'll go to an exhibition and then for coffee. I'll continue watching that TV series after work on Tuesday. And I'll take a relaxing bath when I come home on Thursday.

Exercise

A long walk on Sunday with my husband. A brisk walk during lunch on Wednesday.

Mindfulness

I'll do the "Body Scanning" with my partner tonight and the "Breathing Anchor" tomorrow after work.

CHAPTER 7 EXPANDED SECTION

If you want to improve your communication and relationship skills and understand your emotions better, then the expanded section of this chapter is for you. To start with, we'll take a closer look at what makes communication in a relationship work. We'll also give you further insights into emotions. Understanding your emotions is an essential skill when it comes to building healthy relationships.

Listening Before Problem Solving

We all need to vent some difficult emotions sometimes. Perhaps we need to feel seen and understood, or need to feel accepted, and talking about the matter can be a way of connecting with our emotion.

Often the listener means well but makes things worse by taking on the role of problem solver instead of just affirming our feelings. This can make us feel steamrollered, even if the person we're talking to has only the best of intentions.

Here's an example to show you what we mean. Person A comes home to person B after a hard day at work, and all A wants to do is tell B about her difficult day and get a little affirmation.

Person A: Arrgh! What a day I've had! I had so much I wanted to do, and I didn't even get around to doing half of it! And then in the middle of everything my boss comes in and dumps even more stuff on my desk!

Person B: But I've told you that you need to talk to your boss. You've got to start saying no to things! I also think you have to start writing proper to-do notes every day and prioritizing what's most important. Stick them on your computer. And then you've got to sit down with your boss and get this situation sorted out.

Person A: You just don't get it!

The one who's already at home, person B, means well but puts on the problem-solver's hat and tries to help matters by suggesting what person A can do about it. This probably doesn't make tired person A feel particularly affirmed in her/his feelings. It would have been better if person B had just acknowledged what person A was going through without donning the problem-solver's hat (at least in this moment) and just accepted person A's feelings. Let's try again:

Person A: Arrgh! What a day I've had! I had so much I wanted to do, and I didn't even get around to doing half of it! And then in the middle of everything my boss comes in and dumps even more stuff on my desk!

Person B: Wow, sounds like a pretty tough day. And it's not the first time this week you've said that work is piling up on you. Should we put our heads together and think about what you could do about it? Or do you just want to talk about it later?

Person A: Let's talk about it another time. How about fixing dinner and then we can watch a movie?

Sometimes we don't need a solution; some situations and feelings are a part of life and don't need to be problem solved in that minute, if at all. Say that someone tells us a close friend has just died. A simple and empathetic "I'm sorry to hear that; please let me know if I can do anything" is often a helpful response, and sometimes nothing more needs to be said. Or if a friend tells you that he has just broken up with his long-standing partner, all that's needed is affirmation and emotional connection: "How are you doing? Do you want to talk about it?"

Nurturing Relationships

Most of us have a relationship that has some degree of friction or irritation, like an old conflict that needs resolution or something unsaid that needs saying. Maybe something needs fixing or changing for the relationship to feel more functional and rewarding. Sometimes we wait for the other person to take the initiative, or we simply try to avoid thinking about it. But at the same time, maybe, deep down, we feel a bit sad about having such unresolved conflicts with friends or family members.

Think about your relationships. Is there anything you can do to nurture some of them a little better? We often have limited opportunities to control what other people do, but almost endless opportunities when it comes to what *we* say or do. You have a lot of control over how you develop a relationship with someone. Remember, not making a decision to take control or change is, itself, also a decision.

Do you have a relationship in which you feel that something needs to be said or done? It doesn't have to be about a conflict; it can be a matter of drawing attention to the fact that you don't meet someone as often as you want to anymore, or of finally thanking or showing your appreciation to someone. Your approach to handling these situations will be slightly different depending on whether it means working through a conflict or just showing a little TLC. We'll take these two situations in turn.

EXERCISE: A RELATIONSHIP WITH AN ACTIVE CONFLICT

This exercise is designed to help when you're in conflict with someone and want your relationship to work better.

Person's name and their relationship to you: _____

Why are you disappointed, angry, or irritated with this person?

_____

_____

_____

_____

How has this conflict affected you?

_____

_____

_____

_____

What has the person done or not done to contribute to the conflict or prevent it from being resolved?

_____

_____

_____

_____

What have you done or not done to contribute to the conflict or prevent it from being resolved?

_____

_____

_____

_____

If you were to say or do something in this relationship, what would be the best way of going about it? Could you put it in a I-message?

_____

_____

_____

_____

When you think about something you could do or say, do any conceivable obstacles appear to block your way?

_____

_____

_____

_____

EXERCISE: A RELATIONSHIP WITH NO DIRECT CONFLICT THAT COULD USE A LITTLE TLC

Person's name and their relationship to you: _____

If you decide to do nothing at all and just carry on as usual, how do you think it will affect your relationship in the long run?

_____

_____

_____

_____

If you were to say or do something to improve this relationship, what would it be?

_____

_____

_____

_____

If, in some magical way, this relationship worked really well, what would you get out of it? What would it mean to you and what would it add to your life?

_____

_____

_____

_____

Now try the following:

1. Imagine the person sitting in front of you.

2. Read aloud what you've written as if you were saying it to his or her face.

How did that feel?

If you were to actually say all this to the person in question, would it eventually improve your relationship? If you decide that this is what you want to say, what would be the most effective way of saying it? Face to face? On the phone? By mail or email? By text message? Another way?

Neuroscience Research in Social Relationships and Mental/Physical Balance

We've all felt how soothing and relaxing it can be to be with friends while we're going through a bad patch. Researchers have studied the beneficial health effects of social support and found that a lack of intimate relationships is associated with an increased risk of mental and physical ill health, even premature death (Holt-Lunstad, Smith, & Layton, 2010). Naturally, the brain plays an important part in how loneliness affects the body, but recently scientists have gained a deeper understanding of the mechanisms behind how social support promotes physical and mental well-being. Several studies show that prolonged social isolation stimulates the secretion of stress hormones and the nervous system's fight-or-flight response (Cacioppo, Cacioppo, Capitanio, & Cole, 2015), and that the degree of perceived loneliness affects how genes are switched on or off, which can have important impacts on our health and well-being.

One American research team's study (Cole et al., 2015) found that people who experienced a high degree of loneliness had not only systemic indicators of a high level of stress but also more activity in genes that led to harmful inflammation (which is bad for us), while genes associated with fighting virus infections were less active (which is not helpful to us). To ascertain whether this pattern of gene activation was a cause or consequence of loneliness, they divided apes into groups that lived with different degrees of social support and security for a few weeks. Similar to what they had seen in humans, the researchers found that the loneliest apes showed an increase in stress hormones and genetic activity related to a compromised immune system, and thus a higher risk of inflammation. They were even able to show that loneliness impaired the apes' ability to resist viral infections. All these findings indicate that loneliness is a direct cause of higher stress and that caring for and nurturing social relationships plays a crucial part in achieving physical and mental balance, even down to a biogenetic level.

Verbalize Your Emotions

We'll now look a little more closely at emotions. Relationships—especially those that aren't working as well as they could—normally evoke very strong emotions for both parties. When we name our emotions, many things happen. The brain likes predictability and is most at ease when it knows what's going on. This faculty has increased our chances of survival. Imagine a Stone Age person standing outside the cave observing the vague outline of another person a little way off. A wave of fear washes over him and he has to decide: friend or foe? If it's a friend, it can mean that food's on the way; if it's a foe, it can mean death. This is no time for dithering or hesitation. If the caveman decides to think positively and takes the figure to be a friend, it could be a fatal mistake. To decide that it's a foe and to hide away in the cave is the safer bet. That kind of fearful response can be made again and again without its having life-threatening consequences.

Our brains hate the uncertainty that comes with not knowing how to handle the input from our five senses. And this applies just as much to our emotions. When we don't know what we're feeling, it's harder to accept the emotion and move on, and we can become tangled up in a nebulous web of emotions. When the part of the brain that experiences strong emotions is activated, we more easily fall victim to them.

But when we put a name to the emotions, we activate parts of the brain that can dampen the reactivity and the fight-or-flight response. So it could be useful to get some training in putting names to emotions, as it makes it easier to relate to and act on them; it makes us more mindful of them (e.g., Etkin, Büchel, & Gross, 2015).

A good start is to compile a list of different emotions that you can consult when you experience an uncertain feeling. You can find such a list in the appendix and at http://www.newharbinger .com/41283. Putting names to emotions can be particularly helpful in these ambiguous situations:

- *In times of hardship.* When life seems really tough and we experience strong emotions and thoughts, it can be helpful to put words to what we're feeling. This can facilitate understanding and acceptance—acceptance of what's on the inside, not on the outside. Again, we become more mindful.

- *When practicing mindfulness.* An important skill is taking note of what we're experiencing in the moment. By putting words to emotions, we clarify what we're experiencing: "I, here and now, am feeling ..."

- *When we encounter inner obstacles.* If we can put words to the different emotions we feel when encountering inner obstacles in the form of negative thoughts (such as "I can't ..." or "I must not ..."), we can see them more clearly for what they are.

- *When conveying an I-message.* When we need to describe to someone how we react to something she does, it's a great help if we can identify what it is we feel. Putting words to the emotion can clarify for us and the other person just what we're feeling and how we experience the situation.

Emotions That Conceal Other Emotions

Sometimes we can be duped a little into misunderstanding what we really feel. A strong emotion like anger can conceal another emotion we are actually feeling. As we develop, we're shaped by how our family and friends support us in expressing certain emotions. If you grew up in a context where feeling sad was frowned on and the default negative emotion was anger, you might well have learned to translate your sorrow as anger. Over the years this might have become so habitual that you've stopped even noticing the sadness.

When a strong emotion conceals another emotion we're feeling, the overshadowing emotion is referred to as the secondary emotion, and the overshadowed one as the primary emotion. Sometimes the concealment process goes so quickly that we don't have time to register the primary emotion. At other times, almost immediately after feeling the primary emotion, we judge it and the situation in a way that elicits the secondary emotion.

For example: Say you've just found out that you didn't get that manager's job that you'd pinned your hopes on, and your initial emotional response is sadness—this is the primary emotion. Then you start to judge the situation and perhaps rethink: "It *shouldn't* be like this. I'm more competent and have worked here longer than my colleague who got the job. It's not fair!"

After having worked yourself up for a while, your head is just full of anger, the secondary emotion.

You could blindly express the anger by shouting at your boss, but that's probably not the best strategy. A more effective approach would be to explore all your emotions and then think about the smartest way to act.

The primary emotions that are elicited first are unreflective, instinctive responses. If you lose a friend, you feel sad; if someone tries to steal your wallet, you get angry; if someone threatens you, you get scared.

Primary emotions can sometimes be hard to identify, since they can become overshadowed by the secondary emotions they activate. If you are threatened, first you get scared, until the emotion of fear triggers anger and you take action to escape the situation. Secondary emotions can also be activated by learned responses that shape your attitude toward and thoughts about the primary emotion. If you've learned that it's shameful to be sad, shame can eventually overshadow the primary sadness.

Learning to discriminate and open up to your feelings with curiosity, with mindfulness, can be a helpful way to not be totally swept away by them. When you're curious about the feelings and make room for them, you are more free to choose behaviors consistent with your values. Sometimes figuring out the primary emotion a situation triggers can help you get in contact with your needs in that situation.

Anger tends to arise as a secondary emotion concealing other emotions, such as feelings of being hurt, deserted, lonely, or offended. If in a relationship you feel deserted—and instead of talking about it you just get generally grouchy—you risk never having your needs met and ending up struggling with discontent and misunderstanding.

Another example relates to being a parent. As parents we sometimes get angry at a child when really we want to protect the child from danger or some harmful activity or situation. If in this situation we also acknowledge our primary emotion (in this case, fear), we can help the child see the love that motivated our behavior. When a child feels loved and appreciated, she can more easily absorb this information than if she just feels naughty and chastised.

A Life With Healthier Relationships

In this chapter we've shared some of the best methods we know of for making relationships work well. As is the case in all chapters, we encourage you to take the concrete steps in your everyday life that come to mind as you work your way through the book. We hope you'll discover what we've made a case for in this chapter: better working relationships are a great way to a more meaningful and less stressful life. In the next chapter, we'll take a closer look at your relationship to one particular person: yourself.

CHAPTER 8

Being a Good Friend to Yourself

Talk to yourself like you would to someone you love.

—Brené Brown

We're all perfectly imperfect, and that is something that connects us on this journey of life. If we fight this truth, trying to become perfect and flawless, we miss out on life and its joys. Why not accept the beauty that we all share, and accept that we all make mistakes? In your life there's one person you will never get rid of, someone who's with you from the moment you're born to the moment you die—yourself. Your approach to yourself is the single most important thing in your life. The inner voice you direct at yourself is your steady companion. When you are stressed, this voice often gets louder and more harsh and creates unnecessary stress and pain. This chapter focuses on what you can do about that and how to be a better friend to yourself. But first, a check-in and look back at the key points from the previous chapter.

SO HOW ARE YOU DOING?

Did you manage to make a change in communication or relationship with someone? We asked you to look at a relationship and try a new way of communicating. Did you try it out?

If you answered no, what stopped you? Do you have an idea what could help you make the change?

_____

_____

Did you manage to welcome and accept when something stressful happened during the week? We asked you to stop and acknowledge any challenging feelings and thoughts that surfaced. How did it go?

Completed?	Yes	Partly	No

On a scale of 0 to 10, how welcoming and accepting were you to your challenging thoughts and feelings?

0 ——————————— 5 ——————————— 10

Not at all welcoming   Very welcoming

If you actively stopped, acknowledged, and accepted your challenging feelings and thoughts, how did it feel? Was there any difference in how you experienced the event compared with how you normally react?

_____

_____

_____

Circle your responses and rate how recharging each activity was on a scale of 0 (no recovery) to 10 (plenty of recovery).

Activity	Completed?			Recovery, 0 to 10?
Embraced a value	Yes	Partly	No	
Exercised at least twice	Yes	Partly	No	
Did at least two recharging activities	Yes	Partly	No	
Practiced mindfulness at least once	Yes	Partly	No	

External Events That Got in the Way

If you replied "No" for any of these activities, please write down any external events that got in the way of your completing the activity. How could you overcome these obstacles in the future?

Activity	External obstacle	Ideas on how I can deal with this
Embraced a value		
Exercised two times		
Did two recharging activities		
Practiced mindfulness at least once		

Internal Responses That Showed Up

Write down any negative thoughts, emotions, or physical sensations that showed up, and how you approached them, when doing your activities.

Activity	Internal responses (feelings, thoughts, bodily sensations)	Rate how open and allowing you were able to be (1 to 10)
Embraced a value		
Exercised two times		
Did two recharging activities		
Practiced mindfulness at least once		

How Have You Been Embracing Your Values?

How many actions have you taken this past week in the four areas? Bear in mind both quantity and quality. It will help to have your Life Compass in front of you.

What does your Life Compass look like for the past week?

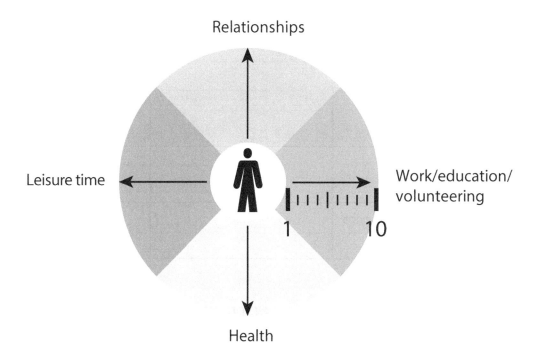

With your Life Compass rating in mind, is there anything you'd like to do more or less of over the coming week? Some area you'd like to give more priority to? Some area that you haven't gotten around to yet? It's best to choose an achievable action, nothing too ambitious.

_____

_____

KEY POINTS FROM CHAPTER 7

The Importance of Calm and Clear Communication

Depending on how we say something, we can create either more understanding or more conflict and separation. We talked about one of the most well-used, effective communication techniques: the I-message. This statement of a feeling always begins with "I." For example, "I feel sad when we argue." Key ingredients of the I-message are telling someone what *you* feel when the person acts in a certain way and how you wish the person would act instead.

Saying No

It can be hard to say no if you're afraid that by doing so you'll be left out or considered boring. It can also be hard if you normally feel that you *should* say yes, for whatever reason. One tip for not feeling forced to say yes to everything is to thank the person for asking you and asking for a little time to think it over.

Asking For Help

When we're feeling stressed we can easily fall into the trap of trying to solve all our problems ourselves and taking on more than we need to. For many people, asking for help can be the key to reducing stress. Letting go and trusting others to take responsibility can be a major challenge, but in the end, asking for help in small steps can eventually be quite liberating.

CORE SECTION: BEING A GOOD FRIEND TO YOURSELF

"So typical of me! I'm the worst person at getting things done on time. I've really got to pull my socks up!"

"I'm far too comfortable; I'm lazy, and I'll have to get my act together if I'm going to make anything of my life. I mean, it's not like I'm particularly talented."

Do you recognize these very self-critical ways of thinking? Sometimes we think the best and quickest way to bring about change is to be hard on ourselves. We're afraid of being lazy and selfish if we prioritize our own needs and show too much kindness and consideration toward ourselves. We can also get hung up on the idea that we have to be strong, independent, and able to cope on our own. But there is growing research evidence of a positive correlation between well-being and self-compassion (e.g.,

Breines et al., 2014; Germer & Neff, 2013; Baer, Lykins, & Peters, 2012; Albertson et al., 2014; Allen & Leary, 2010; Smeets et al., 2014; Kearney et al., 2013; Abaci & Arda, 2013; Heernan et al., 2010; Neff, 2010; and Neff, 2012). When we're kind and forgiving to ourselves, we tend to learn things more easily too. Imagine a little girl trying to learn something difficult. If she is scolded and criticized for her effort, she'll be on her guard. When the part of her brain that deals with fear is activated, it will be harder for her to absorb information and draw on previous experiences. If, on the other hand, she feels appreciated and secure, she will be better able to explore the difficult situation and use more parts of her brain to learn from the new experiences, and she'll be more comfortable with failing and able to improve by learning from those failures. This is also true for adults. There is compelling evidence that praise, appreciation, and acceptance create a conducive context for learning and development (e.g., Baruch-Feldman et al., 2002; Arch et al., 2014), but that isn't always the environment in which we have operated. Our efforts and activities may have been mocked as kids; we may have been bullied for our relative inability to play a particular sport; or we may have grown up with parents who had mental health issues or drug problems, who weren't able to support us with adequate love. Nor is it unusual to grow up with demanding parents for whom nothing is good enough, who cannot relax, take care of themselves, or say no to others. If so, we might well have internalized these behavioral patterns and then impose the same unrealistic expectations, demands, and overly critical evaluations on ourselves. We don't always know why we make such demands of ourselves or why our inner voices are so harsh. But whatever our childhood environment was like, and no matter what we now say to ourselves, we can change. We can still be really good, compassionate friends to ourselves. Being compassionate does not mean thinking positively about ourselves and stopping the harsh words once and for all; rather, it means accepting ourselves just as we are, whatever mood we are in, or whatever thoughts are showing up. The aim of this chapter is to help you to do that.

Your Best Friend and Your Worst Enemy: You

If we take self-criticism seriously—as an accurate evaluation of ourselves—it stresses us, oppresses us, and makes us feel even worse. By cultivating compassion and mindfulness, we can instead activate parts of the brain that inhibit the fight-or-flight response and stimulate the peace-and-quiet system (e.g., Bhasin et al., 2013; Dusek et al., 2008).

We'll soon be looking at how you can train yourself in self-compassion skills, often with the help of mindfulness. This will facilitate well-being in your everyday life and at particularly difficult times. Since the brain is trained to be on the lookout for threats and danger, nurturing this well-being takes practice. We need to work compassionately to discover the more friendly voice in us, as it sometimes is hard to hear above the loud criticism that can build up in our heads.

We All Have Our Inner Hell

Our needs are basically simple and universal. We all want to be acknowledged, affirmed, accepted, and respected. This is one reason why social media has grown so popular. Social media gives us simple, fast access to affirmation from others. The downside, however, is that it also enables us to compare ourselves with others. We get status updates showing us others' polished and manipulated exteriors. When we compare these perfect exteriors with our occasional feelings of sadness, boredom, worries, and inadequacies, we can begin to think that we're unique in harboring these challenging views. "If only I were on a boat trip in the Mediterranean, like Jane and her friends (whose picture received 130 "Likes" on Facebook!), I would be happy." We may begin to feel that our uniquely dull life is the cause of our unpleasant thoughts and feelings. But this is not the case. You can bet that Jane and her friends on that boat carry around their own inner hells (even though they may also have nice tans). Even the most successful people suffer self-doubt and have difficult periods in life. Think of how many beautiful, rich, and famous Hollywood stars are in rehab or have died from substance abuse. We are all vulnerable human beings with the same needs, fears, and self-doubt; we all suffer. It is a human condition, like breathing. If we can accept this state of affairs, we can help manage our expectations and then learn how to handle those difficult thoughts and feelings shared by *everyone* who breathes. As Dr. Brené Brown puts it: "Imperfections are not inadequacies; they are reminders that we're all in this together."

EXERCISE: MY SAFE PLACE

We can strengthen our empathetic, accepting side—that part of us that sees our difficult thoughts and feelings without judgment. In the exercise, we lead you to a safe place inside yourself. We recommend that you listen to the guided audio exercise "My Safe Place" at http://www.newharbinger.com/41283; if you prefer, you can read it here.

The exercise can kindle lovely, positive feelings; it can also elicit sadness. Allow yourself to feel everything you feel, as nonjudgmentally and openheartedly as possible, and to empathize with yourself.

It's best to do this exercise in a peaceful, quiet setting where you won't be disturbed.

1. Start by taking a comfortable seat and then look around the room.

2. Note that you're in a safe place—there is no one to judge you or think anything about you. You can be completely calm in this place. Now close your eyes and picture a place—real or imaginary, past or present—in which you feel calm and safe. Maybe you're alone, maybe you're with someone who makes you feel safe and content. Imagine this situation as vividly as you can.

   What are your surroundings like?

   What time of day or night is it?

Can you see yourself? If so, what do you look like?

If there is anyone else there, what does that person look like?

3. Really explore the feeling of what it's like to be in that safe situation.

4. Allow yourself to accept the sense of security and calm that you associate with the situation. If grief or other emotions pay a call, welcome them too; there's room for them. Allow yourself to experience all the feelings you have and do your best to remain in this place for a while. It is your safe place that always exists inside you and that you can always visit when you feel stress and doubt, such as when you take actions to pursue what gives your life meaning. The exercise is now coming to an end. Picture the physical room you're actually sitting in, and, in your own time, open your eyes.

5. Now answer the following questions.

How did you experience your safe place, and how did you feel when you were there?

_____

_____

_____

_____

What emotions did the exercise arouse? Circle all that apply.

Grief	Rest	Strength	Anger
Security	Acceptance	Freedom	Peace
Joy	Protection	Calm	Love
Other:			

Does the exercise make you think of actual things you can do to be more kind to yourself or any needs you want to start to satisfy more?

_____

_____

_____

_____

Angela's Example

I've realized that I rarely give myself time to sit back and enjoy just being. I really need to drop everything for a while now and then. The best time is when I put on some music I like and listen to it on the sofa.

If you find that your mind is blank or starts to wander and you can't imagine anything, that's fine. Many people find it hard to imagine things and see them in their mind's eye. You might need to do the exercise a few times before your image starts to get clearer. If you were distracted and started to think of something else, try stretching and opening your eyes while doing the exercise. Then have another go.

EXERCISE: FIND YOUR LOVING VOICE

This exercise can help you connect with feelings of willingness and affection toward yourself and others. We recommend that you listen to the guided audio exercise "Find Your Loving Voice" at http://www.newharbinger.com/41283; if you prefer, you can read it here. Choose a place where you won't be disturbed and start whenever you feel ready.

1. Begin by making yourself comfortable and look around the room.

2. Register that it's a safe and secure place. Close your eyes and make contact with your breathing as it flows in and out of your body like waves on a shore.

3. Imagine someone for whom you feel great affection—a child, a parent, or a friend.

4. Ask yourself whether you would still love this person even if the person made a mistake.

5. Imagine that this person feels inadequate and is full of negative, self-critical thoughts. How does this make you feel? Allow yourself to feel your compassion toward this person.

6. Let the image fade.

7. Now think of someone else. It could be a real person, living or dead, or someone you imagine. Have this person represent and convey complete acceptance and unconditional love. Perhaps you are imagining a grandparent, a relative, a teacher, an old acquaintance, or someone you once saw on a movie screen. It could be someone you believe is a symbol of love, a religious figure. It could be your partner, your friend, or a child—any type of person. It could even be an animal. See if you can make the image of this individual, animal, or force (such as the sun) even sharper in your mind. Can you see its face, its loving eyes and smile? Can you see the person or force showing complete acceptance and affection toward you? This person accepts you regardless of what happens, of what you think or feel about yourself. This person sees beyond your negativity, self-criticism, and even failure in pursuing what leads to a life that is vital to you. This

person accepts you, loves you, and is compassionate toward you and what you think and feel, however "bad" that internal response is.

8. Allow the person to continue regarding you with affection and compassion. Allow yourself to be seen with all your shortcomings and with all the negative judgments and feelings that you have about yourself, as you pursue a valued life.

9. Now let the image fade while retaining this feeling of compassion. Can you look back at yourself as a young child, even as a baby? What do you look like? Can you expand your compassion to this little version of yourself who still exists inside you and who still needs your acceptance and compassion?

10. When you feel ready, and in your own time, picture the room you're in and open your eyes. Spend a moment writing your experiences of the exercise down.

11. How did the compassion the person gave you make you feel?

_____

_____

_____

12. How can you draw on that compassion in your daily life? What actual things can you do to be more kind to yourself?

_____

_____

John's Example

This exercise really gave me perspective. I see now how hard I am on myself and how forgiving I am toward others. It's done me good to spend more time with friends who give of their time and who care about me, and to sometimes be fussed over. I'd like to start hanging out more with Matt; he's a good listener.

If you found it hard to visualize pictures in this last exercise you could repeat the first one in the "My Safe Place" exercise a couple of times, until you feel that it comes more naturally. Then you can move on to the "Find Your Loving Voice" exercise. If you were distracted and started to think of something else, try stretching and opening your eyes while doing the exercise. Then try again.

How I'll Be More Kind to Myself

You've now begun training your self-compassion "muscle." For some people this can take time; others connect with their inner voice immediately. If you think that you could benefit from more compassion in your life, we recommend that you do one of these exercises a couple of times a week or more. When we want to change something in our lives it's useful to look at *what we do*, since it's our behavior that we can change—not our thoughts and feelings. So we'd like you to take another look at your Life Compass. See if the exercises highlighted an existing or even new value on your Life Compass—if so, circle that value on your Compass, or add it to your Compass, and write it in the blank that follows. Think about the behaviors associated with this value that you can adopt, even if you have to change something to do so, and write them down on your Life Compass and in this space.

Value: _____

Actions: _____

_____

TAKING ACTION: WHAT YOU CAN DO BEFORE READING THE NEXT CHAPTER

Schedule a day for reading Chapter 9, the final chapter of this book. As always, a week from now would be a good idea. As always, we'll now suggest some meaningful activities you can do before you move on to the next chapter. To begin with, look back at how you rated your actions in your Life Compass at the beginning of this chapter. Is there anything you want to do more or less of and can accomplish? Make a note of those and schedule them into your week. We'd also recommend the following:

- **Embrace a value.** Make time for one value in an area of your choosing. Take at least one concrete step. Pick a small step, something easy to do.

- **Stay open to opportunities to act wisely.** As before, acknowledge the presence of any challenging thoughts and feelings that come up as you work to achieve goals that you value. Try to mindfully note those thoughts, acting mindfully toward them rather than fighting or becoming entangled in them.

- **Be kind to yourself.** Take time for self-care. What concrete behavioral change(s) can you make before the next chapter to be kinder to yourself? It could be what you noted in the "Find Your Loving Voice" exercise or listening to that exercise or the "My Safe Place" exercise again. It could be as simple as reminding yourself what you are grateful for.

- **Exercise.** Schedule one or two (or more) pulse-raising exercise sessions (at minimum, a brisk thirty-minute walk).

- **Mindfulness.** Schedule at least one guided mindfulness exercise from the book's website, http://www.newharbinger.com/41283, and do it.

FOLLOW JOHN AND ANGELA IN THEIR EFFORTS TO LIVE A MORE MEANINGFUL AND BALANCED LIFE

Angela

Embrace a value

I've decided to follow my value of assertiveness and talk to my daughter about not having the time to prioritize helping her prepare a party for friends.

Accept and stay open

I think I've nailed this in many ways in my life now. It seems to come more naturally, and I don't battle with myself as often. I'll continue being accepting and attentive when something difficult crops up or when things don't turn out as I expected.

Being kind to myself

These exercises really aroused something in me. I realize that I rarely do things just for myself. I'm a music lover and miss having it in my life. I'll lie on the sofa listening to music every day this week, just for a short while. I'll also get tickets for a concert that I really want to go to.

Exercise

I'll keep taking walks. I'll also go swimming once this week. I'll ask Debbie if she wants to join me.

Mindfulness

I'll do both the exercises in this chapter; I thought they were great. But it was hard to focus, so I figure I can do them again to practice focusing.

Do you need an extra dose of self-administered love and empathy? Would you like to see which important people have been there for you, and thank them for it? If so, the expanded section of this chapter is for you.

CHAPTER 8 EXPANDED SECTION

If you feel the focus on self-compassion in this chapter has been helpful, you can get a lot out of this expanded section. The exercises here are powerful tools to help you be a better friend to yourself.

EXERCISE: A LOVE LETTER TO YOURSELF

One way of creating self-compassion is to come face to face with your child self. We've all had our fair share of trials and tribulations, some of us more than others. No one's childhood is perfect; chances are all of us have had times when we felt lonely and abandoned, when our need for intimacy—or boundaries—wasn't respected, when nasty things were said to us, or when we just felt left out.

In this exercise, we won't ask you to dig up your most painful or distressing memories. If you know you've been through some really traumatic event and don't feel that you can face the emotions the memory will elicit, we recommend you skip this exercise and move on to the next, "The Good Parent." Or choose a less difficult time in your youth, and write to your young self at that point. Read Angela's letter, which follows, and see if this is something you can manage; if not, that's okay; "The Good Parent" exercise is very useful, in and of itself!

You're now going to write yourself a letter, a letter from your adult self to your childhood or adolescent self—a letter acknowledging your past. It can be written to you at a specific time in your life or be more general. Here's some advice you might like to follow:

- Show your younger self that you can see the challenging thoughts and feelings he or she had and the difficulties he or she was facing.

- Show your younger self that you understand these thoughts and feelings. Tell this child it was okay to think and feel that way just then, given the circumstances.

- Tell your younger self that despite his or her past and doubts, it's still possible to take actions that can help continually create the life your younger self wants to shape and mold.

- Avoid telling your younger self things like "Pull yourself together!" or "You've got to be strong!"

As an example of such a letter before you start, here's what Angela wrote in hers:

Dear, sweet eight-year-old. I can see that things aren't very good for you right now. Your parents are fighting and your mother's really depressed. You're really unhappy and feel so lonely. There's so much you don't understand now, and that's fine. You can't understand everything. But I want you to know that I see you and what you're going through. I'm here for you. I want you to know that things will get better before long. They'll calm down, and you'll get through this difficult time. You're not alone.

I see your strengths. You're sensitive and caring. You see others having a hard time, and you're there for them. You're also sensitive to how things are for your parents.

That's nice. You do your best in all kinds of situations. Lots of people love you, even if that's not always easy to believe at this point. I see that you sometimes feel empty and alone. You feel that you always have to be strong. I understand how tough that is. I'm here for you; you don't always have to be strong. It's okay to be taken care of by someone else sometimes.

I see how hard you try to make others like you. I see how much effort you put into getting your homework right. That's nice. It's useful to you to be like that.

I just want you to know that whatever happens with these things, it's okay. You don't have to do well to be included. You don't have to do well at everything to be you, to be loved. Whatever happens, you're always you and are lovable just as you are.

You can come to me when you need to. I'm always here for you and will never abandon you.

Write your love letter to yourself here (or on a blank sheet of paper):

_____

_____

_____

_____

_____

_____

_____

_____

_____

_____

_____

_____

_____

_____

_____

_____

_____

_____

_____

_____

_____

_____

_____

_____

_____

Note: If you struggle with painful memories that still cause you suffering, you might want to seek professional help with them. Effective treatments for such problems as well as conditions like post-traumatic stress disorder (PTSD) are cognitive behavioral therapy (CBT) and eye movement desensitization and reprocessing (EMDR).

We hope this exercise, "A Love Letter to Yourself," helped you contact emotions, gain a new perspective, and infuse a bit of compassion when relating to your childhood. We now turn to the issue of harsh self-judgment that your mind may be making about your life right now. Self-critical thoughts have a tendency to heighten our arousal and stress levels, so it's helpful to get some new perspectives on those thoughts. This next exercise can help.

We can be very hard on ourselves at times and can start to see our self-critical thoughts as truths. This criticism is our attempt to reprimand or scold our actions, thoughts, lack of motivation, and feelings that we (even unconsciously) have. We may even have learned that such criticism is good for us, because it will motivate us to do what we should do. Endorsing such a self-critical approach is not useful over time, however. The problems with this approach are normally easier to see when we hear others using it on themselves. When we see it in others, we often want to encourage them not to be so hard on themselves. How ironic that we are often very hard on ourselves when we encounter such thoughts and feelings! We are bound to encounter such self-critical thoughts when life throws us curveballs and we suffer the pain of abandonment, criticism, rejection, or humiliation. At these difficult times, we need to be our own best friend and support ourselves; we need to shift from criticizing ourselves to approaching our thoughts, feelings, and even actions with love and acceptance, even if we acknowledge that we should not take such actions again. We can always love ourselves, as we are far greater than any action that we may take, or any critical and cruel thoughts we may have; we are worthy of love and compassion, simply because we exist.

EXERCISE: THE GOOD PARENT

With this exercise, we're going to help you take a more compassionate perspective. To start with, make sure you're in a calm space where you won't be disturbed.

Start by writing down three to five self-critical thoughts that you tend to have.

_____

_____

_____

_____

_____

Now let go of your active focus on these critical thoughts. Think of someone—a child or an adult—toward whom you feel compassion and acceptance. Make your image vivid, and let your affection for this person spread out into your body. If you like, you can shut your eyes and imagine the person as you produce your warm feelings.

Now imagine this child—or this adult as a child—and again create a vivid mental image. See the child in kindergarten, tiny and vulnerable, needing to be seen and accepted. Keep the picture in your mind until it's really clear.

If this child bore your self-criticism—the thoughts you just wrote down—what would you say to the child by way of comfort? Write it down here. Some things to think about while writing:

- Affirm the child's emotions.

- Show compassion by confirming that everyone feels these things.

- Tell the child that he is just fine as he is, no matter what he might think or feel.

- Avoid contradicting the child's thoughts by saying things like "Sure, you're clever!"

- Avoid saying things like "Pull yourself together! You've got to be strong!"

- It's okay to repeat yourself.

The self-critical thoughts and your comforting words in response:

_____

_____

_____

_____

_____

_____

_____

_____

What Angela Wrote:

I feel stupid. *I know how painful it must be to have these thoughts. It's okay; there's nothing wrong with them. Cleverness doesn't come into it. You're you, and that's great. No matter what your feelings and thoughts tell you, you can still find things in life that give you enjoyment and meaning.*

I feel inadequate. *We all sometimes feel that we're inadequate, and that's okay. I know it's horrible to feel like that, but you're not alone. I think you're great just the way you are. Everyone feels inadequate sometimes. Just keep doing what is important to you. I love you the way you are.*

I'm too assertive and talkative. *You're you, and I love you for who you are. We're all different, and no one is better or worse than anyone else. It's okay for you to have these thoughts and feelings. You don't have to give all your attention to them.*

I've got a horrible body. *Having thoughts like that can't be easy. We've all got things we're not happy with. But I think you're lovely as you are. Your value doesn't lie in your body. You deserve to be loved just as you are.*

EXERCISE: UPS AND DOWNS AND THANKS TO SOMEONE WHO'S BEEN THERE FOR YOU

As we ride life's roller coaster, we may discover that we're sitting with someone who's been with us the whole time. Maybe someone who's listened to us when we've needed to offload, or urged us to take that brave step forward. In this exercise, you'll chart the ups and downs of your life over the past ten years. You can then see who's been there for you and will get a chance to thank them.

To get you oriented to the exercise, take a look at Figure 7, the exercise worksheet as completed by John.

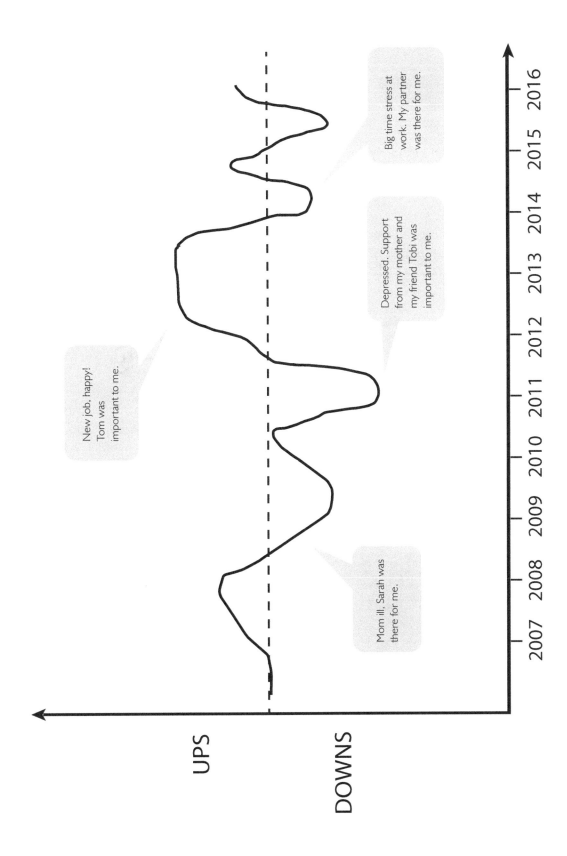

Figure 7: Ups and downs: John's example

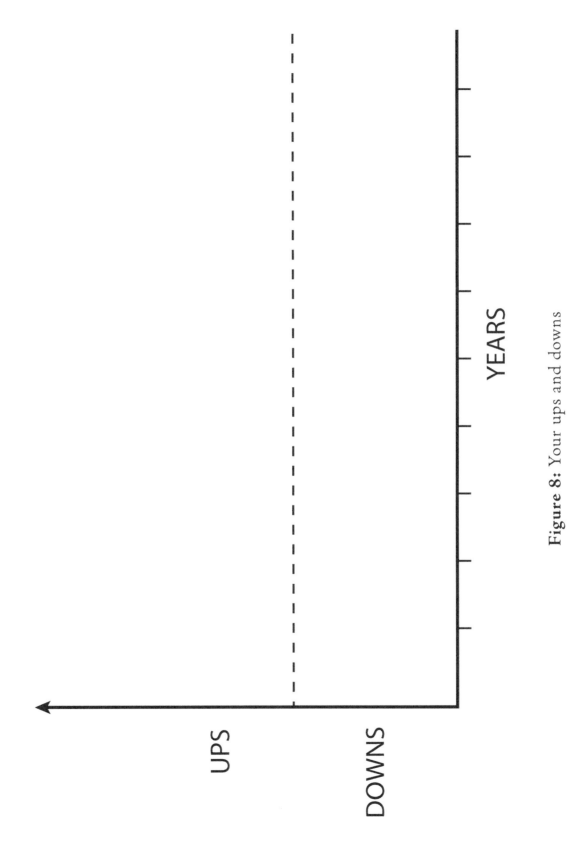

Figure 8: Your ups and downs

1. Using the blank worksheet in Figure 8 (or an "Ups and Downs" worksheet downloaded from http://www.newharbinger.com/41283), mark the years of a decade; this could be the past ten years or an earlier period of your life.

2. Think about the ups and downs, high and low points, that you lived through over this period and depict them with a line. If you don't know exactly when these were or you want to leave some breaks in the curve, that's fine.

3. Write a brief note about what happened during each high and low point.

4. Now think about whether there was a particular person who gave you encouragement or support at these times and write their names at the appropriate points. It might be a person you don't know but who was there for you indirectly, such as the author of a book that helped you. Think freely, but start with people you actually know.

5. Of all the people who were there for you during this time, is there anyone you'd want to especially thank? Maybe you already have and want to do so again? It could be someone who supported you during a rough patch or someone who encouraged you and helped you when times were good. Take this opportunity to thank them. We suggest writing a letter; you can then either read it to the person, print and send it by snail mail, email, or text message, or you could video yourself and send the file to them on your smartphone. (In our experience, people are most touched when the message is read to them in person or by video.)

I'd like to show my appreciation to:

_____

_____

_____

_____

My thank-you letter:

_____

_____

_____

_____

_____

_____

_____

_____

_____

_____

_____

_____

_____

_____

_____

_____

What John wrote:

Dear Sarah,

We were such good friends when we worked together, and I've been thinking about our friendship recently. I hope that you already know this, but I wanted to put it in a letter and read it to you. I just want to let you know how happy I am that you have been a part of my life. It felt as if we were really on the same wavelength, and I'm sure we still are! I loved being with you, as you put me at ease and I could be myself. Everything I said made sense to you; you always tried to understand me, and I never had to feel ashamed of anything I did or said. I miss not having you in my life. You're really special to me. It makes me particularly happy to think of the time when Mom was sick and in the hospital. You were a rock for me then, a stable point in my life and one of the few people I felt I could really talk to. When I think of you I am filled with joy and love. I'm so grateful that you've been my friend. Thank you for being you, because being with you has made me feel fantastic.

Love,

John

Self-Compassion On the Rest of Your Journey

This chapter has been about being a better friend to yourself, about having self-compassion. Think of self-compassion as a muscle that you need to exercise to keep strong. That goes for a lot of the skills and mind-sets that we have covered in this book. In the next chapter—the very last—we'll look ahead to see how what you've learned can be useful for you in your life from now on.

CHAPTER 9

Life from Now On

The only thing that is ultimately real about your journey is the step that you are taking at this moment. That's all there ever is.

—Eckhart Tolle

As you do constantly, every minute of every day, you are now approaching an important part of your life: the next step—or rather, the direction in which you will take your life. But before we discuss this, let's look back at what you've been doing so far.

SO HOW ARE YOU DOING?

When something stressful happened during the week, did you manage to welcome and accept your challenging thoughts and feelings?

Completed? (acknowledged and willingly opened up to challenging feelings and thoughts)	Yes	Partly	No

On a scale of 0 to 10, how welcoming and accepting were you to your challenging thoughts and feelings?

0 ——————————— 5 ——————————— 10

Not at all welcoming   Very welcoming

Was there any difference in how you experienced the event compared with how you normally react?

_____

_____

_____

_____

How Did You Do on Your Other Activities?

Answer these questions and rate how recharging each activity was on a scale of 0 (no recovery) to 10 (plenty of recovery).

Activity	Completed?			Recovery, 0 to 10?
Embraced a value	Yes	Partly	No	
Was kind to myself	Yes	Partly	No	
Exercised at least twice	Yes	Partly	No	
Practiced mindfulness at least once	Yes	Partly	No	

External Events That Got in the Way

If you replied "No" to any of these questions, please describe any external events that got in the way of your completing the activity. How could you overcome these obstacles in the future?

Activity	External obstacle	Ideas on how I can deal with this
Embraced a value		
Was kind to myself		
Exercised at least twice		
Practiced mindfulness once		

Internal Responses That Showed Up

Record any challenging thoughts, emotions, or physical sensations that showed up, and how you approached them, when doing your activities.

Activity	Internal responses (feelings, thoughts, bodily sensations)	Rate how open and allowing you were able to be, 1 to 10
Embraced a value		
Was kind to myself		
Exercised at least twice		
Practiced mindfulness once		

How Have You Been Embracing Your Values the Past Two Months?

You can use the Life Compass in different ways and at different times. For instance, you can use it to sum up the past year or the past week. We, the authors, tend to use it on New Year's Eve to look back at the past year, as it can give some useful hints about resolutions to make for the coming year (if you make new year's resolutions). We suggest that you estimate how many steps you've taken in the past two months in the four areas.

_____

_____

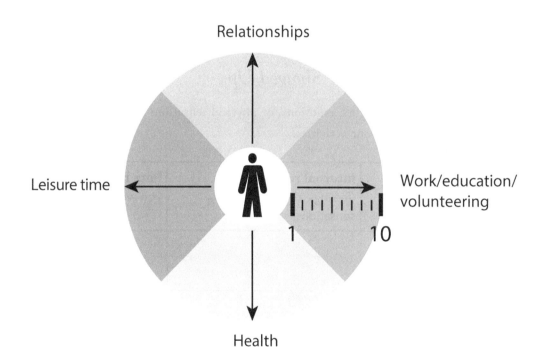

With your Life Compass rating in mind, is there anything you'd want to do more or less of over the coming month? Are there some areas you'd like to give more or less priority to?

KEY POINTS FROM CHAPTER 8

We Each Have Our Own Inner Hell

It's easy for us to believe that other people's lives are better than our own. The truth is, everyone is beset at times by adversity, doubt, and negative thoughts and feelings. Suffering is universal, a shared experience that can bring people together. We're all in the same boat.

Being Your Own Best Friend: Caring in Action

Whatever our baggage, we can learn to take care of ourselves and learn to forgive ourselves for being human and making mistakes. By frequently checking in with our needs and caring for ourselves through actions, we increase our kindness to ourselves.

CORE SECTION: WHAT HAS HAPPENED TO YOUR STRESS LEVELS?

This entire book and the exercises offered are designed to help you make lifestyle changes so you can live your life more in keeping with what's important to you. While reading it, you've no doubt made some changes and tried out different strategies to make your life more meaningful to you—perhaps more rounded in terms of your Life Compass. It's time to again take the stress test that you took at the start of this book to see if you have experienced any changes in your stress levels.

Circle the number for each answer, then add them up to arrive at your score.

In the last month, how often have you …	Never	Almost never	Sometimes	Fairly often	Very often
… been upset because of something that happened unexpectedly?	0	1	2	3	4
… felt that you were unable to control the important things in your life?	0	1	2	3	4
… felt nervous and stressed?	0	1	2	3	4
… felt confident about your ability to handle your personal problems?	4	3	2	1	0
… felt that things were going your way?	4	3	2	1	0

… found that you could not cope with all the things that you had to do?	0	I	2	3	4
… been able to control irritations in your life?	4	3	2	I	0
… felt that you were on top of things?	4	3	2	I	0
… been angered because of things that were outside of your control?	0	I	2	3	4
… felt difficulties were piling up so high that you could not overcome them?	0	I	2	3	4

Interpreting Your Answers

You're the expert on you. Only you can tell how stressed out you really are. Your experience is key. If you like, you can compare your score to the scores of thousands of others who have taken this test (Chan & La Greca, 2013) to determine what category you may fall into: low, average, or high stress (Cohen & Janicki-Deverts, 2012). If your total score is 0 to 7, your stress level is rather low—stress is not a big problem for you right now. Still, you might find continuing the strategies in this book helpful in living a vital life and in preventing future problems! If your score is 8 to 20, you probably have moderate stress problems in your daily life—you definitely would benefit from continuing or even increasing the activities recommended in this book. If your score is 20 or higher, you are most likely suffering from serious stress problems and would probably benefit greatly from following the advice in this book. In addition, we suggest that you consider consulting a professional, such as your general practitioner or a therapist. Remember, the exercises in this book can complement the work a therapist might do with you.

I'm Just as Stressed as Before, If Not More Stressed

There can be many causes of stress: stage of life, time of year, or personal circumstances, to name but a few. Just because your stress levels are at least as high as they were last time you did the test doesn't mean the changes you've made have been in vain or your insights are worthless. Sometimes we rate our stress levels higher simply because our attention has been drawn to the stress we previously weren't aware of. The exercises in this book can help you deal with the stress you were unaware of or were trying to avoid. So there is some internal work you can do, and perhaps some external steps you can take as well. Think about what you can do with situations in your life that are counter to items you've identified in your Life Compass. Can you change them, stop them, or take a different view of them? You have the power to take action in your life! If you feel that you've not been able to follow the advice we've given you in this book, you might want to think about speaking to a professional who offers a CBT approach.

I'm Less Stressed Than Before

Congratulations; that's great news! You've probably made good use of the exercises and advice in this book. You've made changes on several levels to bring better balance to your life. Stress levels can also be affected by life circumstances, so it could be that life is going quite smoothly for you at the moment—and perhaps you've taken steps to make this happen! This is good, so seize the opportunity to make use of the balance you've achieved. Keep using the strategies and attitudes that you find helpful, and don't forget to continue to take actions that address your Life Compass.

Creating a Meaningful Life

When have you felt vital and alive? What were you doing? How about when you felt isolated and unhappy—what were you doing at those points? What do these experiences tell you about what you value in different areas of your life, and what steps you need to take to live out those values over the next week, the coming month, and even the coming year? Ultimately, what actions are you willing to take to continue to shape the life that gives you meaning? Are you willing to accept the stress and doubts that it will take to create that meaning? We invite you to ask yourself these questions about what you want to achieve, what you want to stand for, what qualities you want to explore and express, and what these actions will say about the purpose you are representing.

What I want my life to be about _____

_____

_____

Angela's Example

To spread love and be mindful.

John's Example

To live with an inquisitive, open, nonjudgmental mind.

When we want to make life changes, we can look at them as a chain, linked together in different ways (see Figure 9):

■ We can start to reflect on our own overarching *values*, and let them inform our *goals*, *subgoals*, and concrete *actions*, or

■ We can start by doing small, everyday things differently. Small *actions* lead to *subgoals* and *goals* in keeping with the *values* that we consider important. As they put it in the 1970 Christmas TV special *Santa Claus Is Comin' to Town*, all you have to do is keep putting one foot in front of the other, and before long you'll be walking out the door.

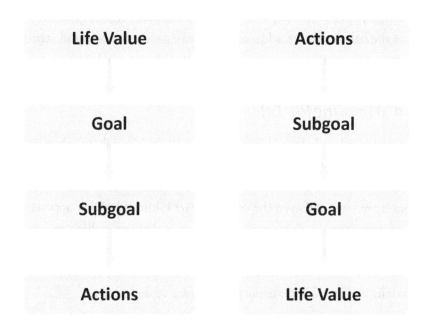

Figure 9: Chain of life changes

We'll soon be looking at the first kind of chain, in which you start with an overarching area and value. But first we'd like to remind you that goals are set and achieved most effectively if they are specific, time-bound, quantifiable, and realistic.

■ *Specific* goals are concrete and self-contained. A nonspecific goal might be "I want more time to myself." A specific and better formulation would be: "I'll take a walk twice a week at lunch."

■ *Time-bound* means the goal can be planned for a certain time. A non-time-bound goal might be "I'll talk to my boss about my workload." A time-bound goal would be "I'll talk to my boss about my workload after Thursday's meeting."

■ *Quantifiable* means the goal can be measured, so you can tell whether you've attained it. A nonquantifiable goal might be "I want to be a better colleague." A quantifiable goal would be "I want to meet my colleagues more often and have lunch with them at least once a week to discuss how work is coming along."

■ *Realistic* goals are not too ambitious or unattainable and can be achieved within a realistic time frame. A nonrealistic goal for someone with a full-time job and young children might be "I'll train at the gym five times a week and have a nice, long uninterrupted breakfast every day." Unrealistic goals like this just lead to failure and condition us to give up the idea of having goals altogether. A realistic goal would be "I'll train once a week and have a nice, unhurried breakfast at work with a colleague once a month."

One last thing to remember is not to set a "dead man's goal"—that is, to aim at something that a corpse would have a better chance of attaining than you would. For example, a dead man is much better than you are at not eating ice cream or not feeling worried or sad. Instead, you can ask yourself: "If I stopped doing all these things, what would I do instead?" In other words, a dead man's goal is about negatives—*not* being this or *not* doing that—which isn't very helpful when setting achievable goals.

EXERCISE: WHAT YOU WANT TO HAVE ACHIEVED WITHIN THE YEAR

You'll now use Figure 10, "The Meaning of My Life" to set out what will be important for you in the coming year or years, consistent with your Life Compass. If you like, you can print out the figure on the book's website, http://www.newharbinger.com/41283. Make a plan for as many years as you like, but we advise between one and five.

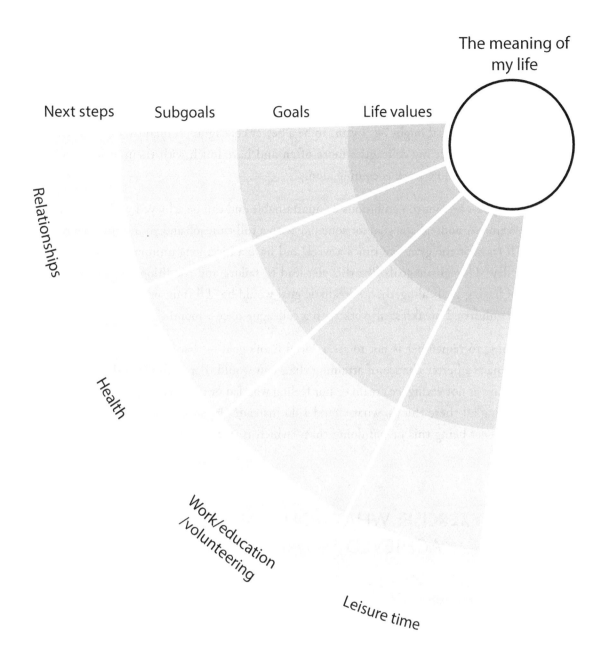

Figure 10: The Meaning of My Life

In the empty circle headed "The meaning of my life," you can write what you just wrote under the heading "What I want my life to be about."

Then choose an area (health, work/education/volunteering, leisure time, relationships) in which you feel a real need for change. The time span here is at least for the year ahead—more if you think it necessary. If you want, you can let your "meaning of your life" inspire you to identify the right area.

Is there a value in this area that is especially important to you? Or do you want to formulate a new value here? Write it on the figure under "Life values."

_____

_____

_____

Using the value you've chosen, can you name one or more related, concrete goals that you'd like to have achieved in a year's time (or more)? Add it to the figure under "Goals" and/or write them here. Remember our earlier advice on setting goals.

_____

_____

_____

How will this goal help you work toward your value? Why is it important? What positive changes could it bring to your life?

_____

_____

_____

It's useful to break down goals into subgoals. Write the subgoals on the diagram or here. What subgoals do you want to set up toward reaching your goal?

_____

_____

_____

_____

_____

_____

_____

_____

Finally, identify the actual next steps you need to take, starting today (or at least tomorrow), that will help you achieve one of the goals or subgoals you have identified. Maybe you need to look something up online, phone a friend, or do something else relatively small. Do make your subgoals small enough so that you can achieve them; reaching your subgoals and goals should not be a race. Moving toward your values is certainly not a race, because you can never achieve values once and for all (for example, you can't go to your son's football match one day and then you'll forever be a good dad—you have to keep at it). So be realistic in what you plan to achieve!

Given this advice, what things could you do in the coming hour or days that will help you achieve one of your subgoals or goals? Note them here or add them to the figure under "Next steps."

_____

_____

_____

_____

_____

_____

_____

_____

Now that you've identified what you could do, record it in your diary or journal, ideally for within the coming week.

If you want to set up goals and subgoals in more areas, which we suggest you do, you can keep adding to the figure. It's a good idea to put the figure up somewhere where you'll see it, and to tell your friends or partner about what you intend to achieve—remember, telling someone your goals motivates you to complete them.

John's Example

What is meaningful to me: *To live with an inquisitive, open mind.*

Area in my Life Compass: *Relationships.*

Value: *Being courageous and honest.*

Goal for the next year: *I want to have traveled somewhere with my two closest friends, Andy and Mia.*

Why important: *Because they give my life real meaning. I'd like to prioritize spending time with them, as it could bring us even closer together. I also think I'd be happier and more secure if we had a deeper relationship.*

Subgoals: *To contact both of them, find a date we can all make using some online calendar app, and arrange to meet so we can discuss where to go and make plans.*

Next step: *Email Mia and Andy to see if they're interested.*

WHAT TO TAKE WITH YOU

We're now reaching the end of the book. The idea was for you to try out its many tips and techniques and to wait until the end before evaluating what works and what doesn't work for you right now. You can now decide what you think will help you as you move on in life. We hope you've identified at least one thing that could help you pursue a meaningful life by achieving your subgoals and goals. So we'll now review the book's key points about handling stress and give you some more general tips for the future. We'd like you to mark the tips or techniques you want to take with you. And—we repeat—don't forget to schedule concrete steps to take. *It's by taking concrete steps, or actions, that you change your life!* Mindfulness and other skills may help you take these actions (for example, by reducing your stress levels), but it's the action that makes all the difference.

Read through the following key points, and as you read through, circle headings you like, that are relevant to you, and that you want to take with you. Next, in the "Useful Strategies" section you can check the relevant ones and also note how you'll take action. We suggest you download this summary and action sheet from the book's website, http://www.newharbinger.com/41283, and keep it where you easily can see it as a reminder.

Take Note of When You're Stressed

Being under stress for a long time can accustom us to a high level of activity or different stress behaviors, and we end up becoming unaware that we're stressed. The first step toward handling stress is becoming aware of how it affects your body, your mood, your mind, and your behavior. Write a list of your personal indicators and stick it on the fridge or give it to a partner or close friend as reminders for when you're stressed. You can also download and use a Stress Journal to keep track of the daily hassles that trigger your stress. You'll find it on the website for the book, http://www.newharbinger.com/41283.

Be Prepared for Stress at Times of Crisis

Major life changes, even those that we welcome, often create stress—no matter how much we've been longing to move, have a child, or start a new job. When a life event has already occurred, draw up a recovery plan, ask for help, delegate, and offload. When a life change is on its way, schedule acceptance and recovery practices *before* it starts. Reserve time in your diary, and don't book too many commitments. If you have time to arrange restorative activities with others, your plans are more likely to come to fruition.

Plan for Recovery

Short-term stress is vital to life and harmless. More chronic, uninterrupted stress, however, can cause all manner of physical and psychological problems. Always make sure to schedule restorative activities, such as mindfulness exercises and making plans driven by your Life Compass. Some of these activities may require hours, if not days, but you can always set yourself subgoals to help you along your journey toward recovery. Of course, planning activities around your Life Compass may help you minimize or maybe even avoid long-term stress.

Get Regular Exercise

Exercise is one of the most effective ways of handling stress. When we exercise, we mitigate the effects of stress hormones on the brain and body. So make sure to schedule time for it. Remember, doing a specific type of exercise might be consistent with other Life Compass values; for example, going to a gym may provide you with contact with other people that a solitary run won't offer.

Take Short Breaks

When you take short breaks, you reduce your total stress. Every little break helps bring your life into better balance in the long run. Take regular short breaks, breathe deeply three times, drop your shoulders, have a cup of tea or water, and stop what you're doing for a few seconds. Schedule or set a reminder for these breaks. They're worth doing regularly.

Practice Mindfulness to Recover from a Stressed Mind

In today's society, we have a lot to think about and a lot of information to process. Our constant stream of thoughts can stress us. However, with an open, accepting attitude, we can let thoughts come and go and practice the ability to return to the moment. Practice mindfulness regularly, with or without our guided exercises. You can stream or download all the book's exercises for free from http://www.newharbinger.com/41283. There is also a wealth of free apps to explore, such as "Insight Timer." If you want to delve more deeply into mindfulness, consider taking a course in mindfulness-based cognitive therapy (MBCT) or mindfulness-based stress reduction (MBSR) at a yoga center, through external university centers, or other places.

Get Proper Sleep

Insomnia, stress, and other psychological problems are closely related. There are many aids for a good night's sleep, including giving yourself enough time to get ready for bed, banishing TV and electronic devices from the bedroom, and avoiding stimulating activities just before bedtime. Prioritizing sleep is surprisingly effective at making you feel better and reducing stress. Give it a try: set up a strategy based on the tips in this book and follow it for a couple of weeks to see if you start sleeping better (see Chapter 1 for strategies). If you have serious problems sleeping, you should contact a doctor and maybe find a CBT course or self-help book that directly targets sleep problems, such as *The Sleep Book: How to Sleep Well Every Night* by sleep expert Dr. Guy Meadows (2014).

Be True to Your Values

When we're stressed, we tend to do more of the "shoulds" and "musts" and less of what would be restorative and possibly most meaningful to us. This is why we've emphasized consulting your Life Compass so often. A loss of meaningful direction in life makes recovery difficult and can cause a kind of existential stress—"What is life about? Why should I live? I don't need to suffer through this grinding existence." The Life Compass can give you feedback on how you live your life and what you need to prioritize to live more in line with your values, which will give your life meaning and reduce stress. You are most likely to succeed in this endeavor if you focus on your own role and what you can do yourself in working on the goals associated with your Life Compass. So return regularly to your Life Compass to help you keep on a meaningful track in your daily life, and talk about it, or your goals, with your friends or family. Schedule activities in keeping with your Life Compass, and be sure to take a long look at the values in it every year or so, perhaps at the new year.

Don't Put Off or Avoid Problems; Solve Them!

We have the power to change many things that cause us stress, but they can be emotionally difficult to face. If we take on the discomfort or distress promptly, we can prevent its growing even worse and eventually learn to work through that discomfort, which helps us take better care of ourselves. One important step toward solving a problem is to define it. So when encountering a stressful problem, print out a problem-solving form (see Chapter 4), download one from http://www.newharbinger.com/41283, or use a blank sheet of paper—and describe it in as much detail as possible. You can use this definition to think up different creative solutions without judging them. Then choose a workable solution that is consistent with your values, and make plans for how and when you're going to implement it (perhaps in stages or over time).

To Accept the Inevitable, Accept Your Feelings

Much of the stress we experience in life is caused by some kind of internal struggle. We think there's something wrong *because* we have challenging feelings. Sometimes we just need to be mindful and accept those feelings—opening up to the discomfort and pain that are an inevitable part of life. Other times those negative feelings are red flags indicating that something is wrong in our life. Acceptance is about feeling what you're already feeling and holding it in your open hand without judging yourself. It's good to keep taking note of when you judge yourself or engage in some internal struggle about what already *is* or has occurred. If the bus is late, if you make a mistake, or if you encounter a major crisis, can you welcome your feelings with openness and acceptance? By doing so, you have more space to think about how you can overcome or move through the situations that are causing your pain. Avoiding that pain, however, is unlikely to help you solve a problem in your life.

Challenge Your Avoiding or Performing Self

Many of our habits are counterproductive. We want to be loved just for being who we are, yet we still sometimes believe we have to do everything perfectly to deserve love. When we practice doing the opposite of what we automatically think we "should" or "must" do, we learn that the world doesn't fall apart, we become more true to our own values, and we are typically more appealing to other people—maybe not the people we feel we "should" be friends with, but people who share our values and who can appreciate us for who we actually are. Thus, we not only reduce our stress but also live a more vibrant and meaningful life. Of course, when we change or do something different from our usual habits, we often meet resistance, and the people around us might still expect us to say yes to everything and, in effect, act in the same way as usual. If this happens, you need to bring a healthy dose of acceptance and willingness to the discomfort that comes from failing to meet other people's expectations, as well as the stress of doing something new and differently. During this process, be sure to use the resources you have: discuss things with your closest family and friends. Use I-messages to tell people what you want or why you're doing some things differently.

The Course of Life Isn't Always Smooth; Hurdles Are Inevitable

From an ACT perspective, it's better to deal with hurdles by picking them up and bringing them with you. In other words, when you encounter thoughts or feelings that could obstruct you, see if you can accept their presence without a struggle and without buying into them. Thoughts are thoughts, feelings are feelings. If you are moving toward a goal, or even just relaxing (and self-care is a value for most people!), make yourself aware of the thoughts you have; tell yourself, "I'm thinking [whatever]," and then take another step toward what's important to you. Welcome and accept the challenging feelings that come then, but don't take these as truths, either; also, don't let them bully you into engaging with them. They want attention, and while you need to acknowledge them, you don't have to enter into a dialogue with them. So you *can* take a different approach to your thoughts and feelings. Make room for them, thank your brain for being so active—and then take another step in the direction in which you wish to go.

Communicate What You're Thinking and Feeling

Conflict can easily flare up because we think that others should understand our thoughts and feelings in response to things they do. But it's unlikely that your partner and friends are mind readers; you need to communicate clearly if you're going to effect any change. (Even we psychologists aren't mind readers!) Use I-messages to increase your chances of being understood. Key ingredients of the I-message are telling people what you *feel* when they do a certain thing in a certain way, and explaining what you wish they might do instead. Avoid (1) using the words "never" and "always," (2) digging up old grievances, and (3) accusing the person of "being" something (for example, "You're as lazy as a …"—these pejoratives are generally not accurate, anyway). It's also a good idea to teach this technique, in a kind and thoughtful way, to your partner and friends to make your relationships less needlessly confrontational.

Say No to Things You Don't Want

When you're asked to do something, it can be hard to say no, either for fear of being excluded or considered boring or difficult, or out of a desire to always do the right thing or to please others. We suggest you refer back to your Life Compass and ask yourself whether saying yes is in keeping with what's important to you. You can usually ask for a little time to think about it, and if it is a work situation you can also convey your other commitments. By saying no, you can also keep your yes for the things you truly want in your life. Try practicing this with small requests—and, of course, plan how, when, and to what you're going to say no. Also, on a practical level, remember that sometimes if you plan to say no, because you don't have the time, you can often negotiate the timing of something in order to say yes to it, or you can offer something you *can* do instead. The key is *flexibility* in how you respond, but saying no must always be one of your options.

Ask for Help

For many, part of the negative stress problem is that we tend to want to do everything ourselves and take on responsibility for more than we have to. After a while, others expect this of us, and our taking responsibility becomes habitual. Asking for help can be the key to reducing stress. But letting go of the reins and letting others take over can be a major challenge. Asking for help, step by step, can be liberating! Try starting with something you're confident you can get help with if you ask. The opportunity to help makes many people feel important and competent. This can strengthen the bond between you. In the world of work, asking for help, often called delegating, is a key skill for any top-flight leader; lacking the time, expertise, or perspective of some of their employees, they must ask for help to succeed—and this makes their employees feel valued and motivated.

Practice Everyday Mindfulness—It Can Lower Your Stress Levels

When we're present in the here and now, most problems seem to shrink a little. "Right now" is rarely as unpleasant as the *idea of* what it could be. Studies show that as much as 85 percent of what we worry about never happens. And when something does happen, we manage the situation better than we had imagined we would. Make a habit of stopping to notice where you are and what you're seeing, hearing, and feeling. Use pleasurable moments to be mindful in—why not take advantage of a good feeling? Schedule or set a reminder for times to be mindful.

Be Kind and Forgiving to Yourself

Whatever your experiences, you can practice speaking to yourself more kindly. In much the same way that we can be our own worst enemy, we can also be our own best friend. Research shows that self-compassion can reduce stress and make us more inclined to deal with problems. Self-compassion also makes us better at seeing other people's pain. Practice self-compassion by creating safe places you can return to, either internally or externally, such as with friends who give you security, comfort, or acknowledgment. You can also strengthen your kind voice by planning things that you do just for your sake, such as treating yourself to a trip somewhere or a brief spell of recovery.

Useful Strategies from
The Mindfulness and Acceptance
Workbook for Stress Reduction

Circle or highlight strategies that you find helpful, as discussed in this book. You can always have this list close at hand as a reminder. Use it to take action when you want to make changes in how you live. You can also print copies of this table at http://www.newharbinger.com/41283.

Strategy	Relevant now? (✓)	How I can take action
Take note of when you're stressed		
Be prepared for stress at times of crisis		
Plan for recovery		
Get regular exercise		
Take short breaks		
Practice mindfulness to ease a stressed mind		

Strategy	Relevant now? (✓)	How I can take action
Make sure to get proper sleep		
Be true to your values		
Solve problems—don't just put them off or avoid them		
Accept your feelings to accept the inevitable		
Challenge your avoiding or performing self		
Get past life's hurdles by taking them along on your journey		
Communicate what you're thinking and feeling		
Say no to things you don't want to do		
Ask for help		
Practice everyday mindfulness—it can lower your stress levels		
Be kind to yourself		

WHEN YOU NOTICE YOU'RE STRESSED

The themes, tips, advice, and strategies you've been considering are particularly important to use when you start to recognize signs of stress. In the first chapter, you wrote down the signals you notice in yourself when you're going through stressful times. These will appear as you go through life; this is normal and healthy. No matter how much you've absorbed what you've gone through in this book or the techniques you've used to handle stress, there will inevitably be times when you feel extremely stressed: the death of a loved one, a family crisis, serious health issues, and so forth. We all face such challenges in life.

Let a little alarm bell ring inside you when you end up in a difficult situation or notice multiple signs of stress in yourself, and remember two things:

- We all go through crises and difficult periods at some points in life. But such times pass, no matter how bleak things might seem.

- You can use the strategies you've learned for counteracting the harmful effects of long-term stress. Make use of what you've just marked in the table of strategies. Remember one key to coping with chronic stress: get some recovery time and a chance to wind down.

You've now spent considerable time and energy on reviewing how you live and creating a life that we hope is more consistent with what you want it to be. Every second you've put into this is an investment in yourself. Be proud! Pat yourself gently and kindly on the back and congratulate yourself. We really hope that you've learned some things you'll find invaluable as you continue on your life's journey, living the values that are meaningful to you (and don't let those little voices in your head distract you from that journey ☺).

Acknowledgments

We wish to thank Neil Betteridge and David Haglund for their help with translations from Swedish into English, and Gil Fronsdal for permission to adapt a guided mindfulness exercise.

Appendix: List of Emotions

Interest/curiosity	Joy	Surprise	Anger	Fear	Sadness	Shame	Hatred	Disgust
Open	Happy	Confused	Frustrated	Terrified	Dispirited	Bad	Numbed	Disai::reeable
Receptive	Euphoric	Indecisive	Livid	Upset	Disappointed	Forlorn	Irritable	Dirty
Friendly	Elated	Shy	Aaaressive	Panic-stricken	Depressed	Worthless	Judgmental	Insu l ted
Focused	Nervous	Insecure	Stubborn	Petrified	Powerless	Gloomy	Superior	Deprecatory
Positive	In love	Irresolute	Rebellious	Threatened	Burdened	Guilty	Deprecatory	Nauseous
Considerate	Positive	Hesitant	Tetchy	Uneasy	Resigned	Humiliated	Disagreeable	
In love	Open	Lost	Jealous	Tormented	Self-critical	Lonely	Censorial	
Charmed	Considerate	Tense	Offended	Horrified	Desperate	Ugly	Critical	
Nervous	Jokey	Stressed	Violated	Disjointed	Alienated	Inadequate	Cruel	
Exploratory	Sweet	Uncomfortable	Critical	Worried	Useless	Stupid		
Inquisitive	Relaxed	Distracted	Furious	Paranoid	Belittled	Jealous		
	Inviting	Baffled	Cruel	Rigid	Stuck	Shutdown		
		Embarrassed	Insulted	Concerned	Lethargic	Embarrassed		
			Shut-down	Tense	Blocked			
				Scared	Closed			
				Empty	Withdrawn			
				Abandoned	Hurt			
				Shut-down	Forlorn			
				Restless	Empty			
				Stressed	Lonely			

References

Abaci, R., & Arda, D. (2013). Relationship between self-compassion and job satisfaction in white collar workers. *Procedia-Social and Behavioral Sciences, 106*, 2241–2247.

Åkerstedt, T., Kecklund, G., Alfredsson, L., & Selen, J. (2007). Predicting long-term sickness absence from sleep and fatigue. *Journal of Sleep Research, 16*, 341–345. doi:10.1111/j.1365–2869.2007.00609.x.

Albertson, E. R., Neff, K. D., & Dill-Shackleford, K. E. (2014). Self-compassion and body dissatisfaction in women: A randomized controlled trial of a brief meditation intervention. *Mindfulness*, 1–11.

Allen, A., & Leary, M. R. (2010). Self-compassion, stress, and coping. *Social and Personality Psychology Compass, 4*(2), 107–118.

Andre-Petersson, L., Hedblad, B., Janzon, L., & Ostergren, P. (2006). Social support and behavior in a stressful situation in relation to myocardial infarction and mortality: Who is at risk? Results from the prospective cohort study "Men born in 1914," Malmö, Sweden. *International Journal of Behavioral Medicine, 13*, 340–347.

Arch, J. J., Brown, K. W., Dean, D. J., Landy, L. N., Brown, K., & Laudenslager, M. L. (2014). Self-compassion training modulates alpha-amylase, heart rate variability, and subjective responses to social evaluative threat in women. *Psychoneuroendocrinology, 42*, 49–58. doi:10.1016/j.psyneuen.2013.12.018.

Arnsten, A. F. (2009). Stress signalling pathways that impair prefrontal cortex structure and function. *Nature Reviews Neuroscience, 10*(6), 410–22. doi:10.1038/nrn2648.

A-Tjak, J. G., Davis, M. L., Morina, N., Powers, M. B., Smits, J. A., & Emmelkamp, P. M. (2015). A meta-analysis of the efficacy of acceptance and commitment therapy for clinically relevant mental and physical health problems. *Psychotherapy and Psychosomatics, 84*(1), 30–36. doi:10.1159/000365764.

Baer, R. A., Lykins, E. L. B., & Peters, J. R. (2012). Mindfulness and self-compassion as predictors of psychological wellbeing in long-term meditators and matched nonmeditators. *Journal of Positive Psychology, 7*(3), 230–238.

Bakker, A. B., & Demerouti, E. (2007). The job demands-resources model: State of the art. *Journal of Managerial Psychology, 22*, 309–328.

Baruch-Feldman, C., Brondolo, E., Ben-Dayan, D., & Schwartz, J. (2002). Sources of social support and burnout, job satisfaction, and productivity. *Journal of Occupational Health Psychology, 7*(1), 84–93.

Baumeister, R. F., Campbell, J. D., Krueger, J. I., & Vohs, K. D. (2003). Does high self-esteem cause better performance, interpersonal success, happiness, or healthier lifestyles? *Psychological Science in the Public Interest, 4*, 1–44. doi:10.1111/1529–1006.01431.

Bhasin, M. K., Dusek, J. A., Chang, B.-H., Joseph, M. G., Denninger, J. W., Fricchione, G. L., & Libermann, T. A. (2013). Relaxation response induces temporal transcriptome changes in energy metabolism, insulin secretion and inflammatory pathways. *PloS One, 8*(5), e62817. doi:10.1371/journal.pone.0062817.

Bond, F. W., & Bunce, D. (2000). Mediators of change in emotion-focused and problem-focused work-site stress management interventions. *Journal of Occupational Health Psychology, 5*(1), 156–163. doi:10.1037/1076–8998.5.1.156.

Breines, J. G., Thoma, M. V, Gianferante, D., Hanlin, L., Chen, X., & Rohleder, N. (2014). Self-compassion as a predictor of interleukin-6 response to acute psychosocial stress. *Brain, Behavior, and Immunity, 37,* 109–14. doi:10.1016/j.bbi.2013.11.006.

Brinkborg, H., Michanek, J., Hesser, H., & Berglund, G. (2011). Acceptance and commitment therapy for the treatment of stress among social workers: A randomized controlled trial. *Behaviour Research and Therapy, 49*(6–7), 389–398. doi:10.1016/j.brat.2011.03.009.

Cacioppo, J. T., Cacioppo, S., Capitanio, J. P., & Cole, S. W. (2015). The neuro-endocrinology of social isolation. *Annual Review of Psychology, 66,* 733–67. doi:10.1146/annurev-psych-010814–015240.

Chan, S. F., & La Greca, A. M. (2013). Perceived Stress Scale (PSS). In *Encyclopedia of Behavioral Medicine* (pp. 1454–1455). New York, NY: Springer. https://doi.org/10.1007/978–1-4419–1005–9_773.

Chase, J. A., Houmanfar, R., Hayes, S. C., Ward, T. A., Viladarga, J. P., & Follette, V. (2013). Values are not just goals: Online ACT-based values training adds to goal setting in improving undergraduate college student performance. *Journal of Contextual Behavioral Science, 2,* 79–94.

Chiesa, A., & Serretti, A. (2009). Mindfulness-based stress reduction for stress management in healthy people: A review and meta-analysis. *Journal of Alternative and Complementary Medicine, 15*(5), 593–600. doi:10.1089/acm.2008.0495.

Cohen, S., & Janicki-Deverts, D. (2012). Who's stressed? Distributions of psychological stress in the United States in probability samples from 1983, 2006, and 2009. *Journal of Applied Social Psychology, 42*(6), 1320–1334. doi:10.1111/j.1559–1816.2012.00900.x.

Cole, S. W., Capitanio, J. P., Chun, K., Arevalo, J. M. G., Ma, J., & Cacioppo, J. T. (2015). Myeloid differentiation architecture of leukocyte transcriptome dynamics in perceived social isolation. *Proceedings of the National Academy of Sciences of the United States of America, 112*(49), 15142–7. doi:10.1073/pnas.1514249112.

Cooney, G. M., Dwan, K., Greig, C. A., Lawlor, D. A., Rimer, J., Waugh, F. R.,…Mead, G. E. (2013). Exercise for depression. *Cochrane Database of Systematic Reviews.* doi:0.1002/14651858.CD004366.pub6.

Cornell, K. (2010). *WebKaizen: Better Faster Cheaper Problem Solving for Business.* Omaha, NE: Prevail Digital Publishing.

Cotman, C. W., Berchtold, N. C., & Christie, L.-A. (2007). Exercise builds brain health: Key roles of growth factor cascades and inflammation. *Trends in Neurosciences, 30*(9), 464–72. doi:10.1016/j.tins.2007.06.011.

Dahl, J., Plumb-Vilardaga, J., Stewart, I., & Lundgren, T. (2009). *The Art and Science of Valuing in Psychotherapy: Helping Clients Discover, Explore, and Commit to Valued Action Using Acceptance and Commitment.* Oakland, CA: New Harbinger.

Davidson, R. J., & McEwen, B. S. (2012). Social influences on neuroplasticity: Stress and interventions to promote well-being. *Nature Neuroscience, 15*(5), 689–95. doi:10.1038/nn.3093.

Dunn, A. L., Trivedi, M. H., Kampert, J. B., Clark, C. G., & Chambliss, H. O. (2005). Exercise treatment for depression: Efficacy and dose response. *American Journal of Preventive Medicine, 28*(1), 1–8. doi:10.1016/j.amepre.2004.09.003.

Dusek, J. A., Out, H. H., Wohlhueter, A. L., Bhasin, M., Zerbini, L. F., Joseph, M. G.,…Libermann, T. A. (2008). Genomic counter-stress changes induced by the relaxation response. *PLoS One, 3*(7), e2576. doi:10.1371/journal.pone.0002576.

Ehrman, J., Gordon, P., Visich, P., & Keteyian, S. (2008). Exercise effective treatment for depression. In *Clinical Exercise Physiology* (2nd ed.). Champaign, IL: Human Kinetics. www.humankinetics.com/ excerpts/ excerpts/exercise-effective-treatment-for-depression.

Eisenberger, N. I., & Cole, S. W. (2012). Social neuroscience and health: Neurophysiological mechanisms linking social ties with physical health. *Nature Neuroscience, 15*(5), 669–74. doi:10.1038/nn.3086.

Etkin, A., Büchel, C., & Gross, J. J. (2015). The neural bases of emotion regulation. *Nature Reviews Neuroscience, 16*(11), 693–700. doi:10.1038/nrn4044.

Fantin, I. (2014). *Applied Problem Solving: Method, Applications, Root Causes, Countermeasures, Poka-Yoke and A 3*. Milan, Italy: CreateSpace.

Flaxman, P. E., & Bond, F. W. (2010a). A randomised worksite comparison of acceptance and commitment therapy and stress inoculation training. *Behaviour Research and Therapy, 48*(8), 816–820. doi:10.1016/j.brat.2010.05.004.

Flaxman, P. E., & Bond, F. W. (2010b). Worksite stress management training: Moderated effects and clinical significance. *Journal of Occupational Health Psychology, 15*(4), 347–358. doi:10.1037/a0020522.

French, K., Golijani-Moghaddama, N., & Schröder, T. (in press). What is the evidence for the efficacy of self-help acceptance and commitment therapy? A systematic review and meta-analysis. *Journal of Contextual Behavioral Science*. (Epub ahead of print). http://dx.doi.org/10.1016/j.jcbs.2017.08.002.

Frögéli, E., Djordjevic, A., Rudman, A., Livheim, F., & Gustavsson P. (2016). A randomized controlled pilot trial of acceptance and commitment training (ACT) for preventing stress-related ill health among future nurses. *Anxiety, Stress, & Coping, 29*(2), 202–18. doi:10.1080/10615806.2015.1025765.

Germer, C. K., & Neff, K. D. (2013). Self-compassion in clinical practice. *Journal of Clinical Psychology, 69*(8), 856–867. doi:10.1002/jclp.22021.

Gillanders, D. T., Sinclair, A. K., MacLean, M., & Jardine, K. (2015). Illness cognitions, cognitive fusion, avoidance and self-compassion as predictors of distress and quality of life in a heterogeneous sample of adults, after cancer. *Journal of Contextual Behavioral Science, 4*, 300–311. http://doi.org/10.1016/j.jcbs.2015.07.003.

Gil-Luciano, B., Ruiz, F. J., Valdivia-Salas, S., & Suárez, J. C. (2016). Promoting psychological flexibility on tolerance tasks: Framing behavior through deictic/hierarchical relations and specifying augmental functions. *Psychological Record, 66*, 1–9.

Gleeson, M., Bishop, N. C., Stensel, D. J., Lindley, M. R., Mastana, S. S., & Nimmo, M. A. (2011). The anti-inflammatory effects of exercise: Mechanisms and implications for the prevention and treatment of disease. *Nature Reviews Immunology, 11*(9), 607–15. doi:10.1038/nri3041.

Hains, A. B., Vu, M. A., Maciejewski, P. K., van Dyck, C. H., Gottron, M., & Arnsten, A. F. (2009). Inhibition of protein kinase C signaling protects prefrontal cortex dendritic spines and cognition from the effects of chronic stress. *Proceedings of the National Academies of Sciences 106*(42), 17957–62. doi:10.1073/pnas.0908563106.

Harris, R. (2008). *The Happiness Trap: Stop Struggling, Start Living*. London, UK: Robinson Publishing.

Harris, R. (2012). *The Reality Slap: Finding Peace and Fulfillment When Life Hurts*. Oakland, CA: New Harbinger.

Hayes, S. C., Strosahl, K. D., & Wilson, K. G. (2012). *Acceptance and Commitment Therapy: The Process and Practice of Mindful Change* (2nd ed.). New York, NY: Guilford Press.

Healy, H-A., Barnes-Holmes, Y., Barnes-Holmes, D., Keogh, C., Luciano, C., & Wilson, K. G. (2008). An experimental test of a cognitive defusion exercise: Coping with negative and positive self-statements. *Psychological Record, 58,* 623–640.

Heernan, M., Grin, M., McNulty, S., & Fitzpatrick, J. J. (2010). Self-compassion and emotional intelligence in nurses. *International Journal of Nursing Practice, 16,* 366–373.

Hofer, P. D., Waadt, M., Aschwanden, R., Milidou, M., Acker, J., Meyer, A. H., Lieb, R., & Gloster, A. T. (in press). Self-help for stress and burnout without therapist contact: An online randomized controlled trial. *Work & Stress.*

Holt-Lunstad, J., Smith, T. B., & Layton, J. B. (2010). Social relationships and mortality risk: A meta-analytic review. *PLoS Med, 7*(7). doi:10.1371/journal.pmed.1000316.

House, J. S., Landis, K. R., & Umberson, D. (1988). Social relationships and health. *Science, 241*(4865), 540–5.

Kabat-Zinn, J. (2005). *Coming to Our Senses: Healing Ourselves and the World through Mindfulness.* New York, NY: Hyperion.

Kearney, D. J., Malte, C. A., McManus, C., Martinez, M. E., Felleman, B., & Simpson, T. L. (2013). Loving kindness meditation for posttraumatic stress disorder: A pilot study. *Journal of Traumatic Stress, 26*(4), 426–434.

Klingberg, T. (2009). *The Overflowing Brain: Information Overload and the Limits of Working Memory.* Oxford, UK: Oxford University Press.

Levin, M. E., Hildebrandt, M., Lillis, J., & Hayes, S. C. (2012). The impact of treatment components suggested by the psychological flexibility model: A meta-analysis of laboratory-based component studies. *Behavior Therapy, 43,* 741–756.

Liston, C., McEwen, B. S., & Casey, B. J. (2009). Psychosocial stress reversibly disrupts prefrontal processing and attentional control. *Proceedings of the National Academy of Sciences of the United States of America, 106*(3), 912–7. doi:10.1073/pnas.0807041106.

Livheim, F., Hayes, L., Ghaderi, A., Magnusdottir, T., Högfeldt, A., Rowse, J.,…Tengström, A. (2015). The effectiveness of acceptance and commitment therapy for adolescent mental health: Swedish and Australian pilot outcomes. *Journal of Child and Family Studies, 214*(4), 1016–1030. doi:10.1007/s10826–014–9912–9.

Lloyd, J., Bond, F. W., & Flaxman, P. E. (2013). Identifying the psychological mechanisms underpinning a cognitive behavioural intervention for emotional burnout. *Work & Stress, 27,* 181–199.

Mayer, R. E. (1992). *Thinking, Problem Solving, Cognition* (2nd ed.). New York, NY: W. H. Freeman.

Meadows, G. (2014). *The Sleep Book: How to Sleep Well Every Night.* London, UK: Orion.

Morin, C. M., Bootzin, R. R., Buysse, D. J., Edinger, J. D., Espie, C. A., & Lichstein, K. L. (2006). Psychological and behavioral treatment of insomnia: Update of the recent evidence (1998–2004). *Sleep, 29*(11), 1398–414. PMID 17162986.

Neff, K. D. (2010). Review of *The Mindful Path to Self-Compassion: Freeing Yourself from Destructive Thoughts and Emotions. British Journal of Psychology, 101,* 179–181.

Neff, K. D. (2012). The science of self-compassion. In C. Germer & R. Siegel (Eds.), *Compassion and Wisdom in Psychotherapy* (pp. 79–92). New York, NY: Guilford Press.

Novick, L. R., & Bassok, M. (2005). Problem solving. In K. J. Holyoak & R. G. Morrison (Eds.), *Cambridge Handbook of Thinking and Reasoning* (pp. 321–349). New York, NY: Cambridge University Press.

O'Leary, K., O'Neill, S., & Dockray, S. (2015). A systematic review of the effects of mindfulness interventions on cortisol. *Journal of Health Psychology, 21*(9), 2108–21. doi:10.1177/1359105315569095.

Öllinger, M., Jones, G., & Knoblich, G. (2008). Investigating the effect of mental set on insight problem solving. *Experimental Psychology, 55*(4), 269–282.

Piazza, J. R., Charles, S. T., Sliwinski, M., Mogle, J., & Almeida, D. M. (2013). Affective reactivity to daily stressors and long-term risk of reporting a chronic health condition. *Annals of Behavioral Medicine, 45*(1), 110–120.

Radley, J. J., Rocher, A. B., Miller, M., Janssen, W. G., Liston, C., Hof, P. R.,…Morrison, J. H. (2006). Repeated stress induces dendritic spine loss in the rat medial prefrontal cortex. *Cerebral Cortex, 16*(3), 313–20. doi:10.1093/cercor/bhi104.

Räsänen, P., Lappalainen, P., Muotka, J., Tolvanen, A., & Lappalainen, R. (2016). An online guided ACT intervention for enhancing the psychological wellbeing of university students: A randomized controlled clinical trial. *Behaviour Research and Therapy, 78*, 30–42. doi:10.1016/j.brat.2016.01.001.

Rethorst, C. D., & Madhukar, H. T. (2013). Evidence-based recommendations for the prescription of exercise for major depressive disorder. *Journal of Psychiatric Practice, 19*(3), 204–12. doi:10.1097/01.pra.0000430504.16952.3e.

Savic, I., Perski, A., & Osika, W. (in press). MRI shows that exhaustion syndrome due to chronic occupational stress is associated with partially reversible cerebral changes. *Cerebral Cortex* (Epub ahead of print). doi:10.1093/cercor/bhw413.

Segerstrom, S. C., & Miller, G. E. (2004). Psychological stress and the human immune system: A meta-analytic study of 30 years of inquiry. *Psychological Bulletin, 130*(4), 601–30. doi:10.1037/0033-2909.130.4.60.

Smeets, E., Neff, K. D., Alberts, H., & Peters, M. (2014). Meeting suffering with kindness: Effects of a brief self-compassion intervention for female college students. *Journal of Clinical Psychology, 70*(9), 794–807. doi:10.1002/jclp.22076.

Taylor, J. B. (2006). *My Stroke of Insight: A Brain Scientist's Personal Journey.* New York, NY: Penguin Group.

Uchino, B. N. (2009). Understanding the links between social support and physical health: A life-span perspective with emphasis on the separability of perceived and received support. *Perspectives on Psychological Science, 4*(3), 236–255.

Van Cauter, E., & Spiegel, K. (1999). Sleep as a mediator of the relationship between socioeconomic status and health: A hypothesis. *Annals of the New York Academy of Sciences, 896*, 254–61. doi:10.1111/j.1749-6632.1999.tb08120.x.

Wang, Y., & Chiew, V. (2010). On the cognitive process of human problem solving. *Cognitive Systems Research, 11*(1), 81–92.

Fredrik Livheim, PhD, is a licensed clinical psychologist in the department of clinical neuroscience at the Karolinska Institutet in Stockholm, Sweden. He has trained more than 1,500 professionals in how to use acceptance and commitment therapy (ACT) in a group format to improve employees' mental health. His research focuses on the use of ACT to reduce stress and help people thrive.

Frank W. Bond, PhD, is professor of psychology and management at Goldsmiths, University of London, where he is also director of the Institute of Management Studies. He has published widely in the areas of ACT and organizational behavior, and the processes that underpin peak performance and well-being in the workplace. He is currently using this interdisciplinary research to help the European Space Agency's manned mission to Mars in the next decade.

Daniel Ek, MS, is a licensed clinical psychologist and mindfulness teacher, with professional experience in stress management. Ek treats patients with stress and chronic fatigue syndrome (CFS) on a daily basis, and trains professionals in how to use ACT in a group format to improve employees' mental health.

Björn Skoggård Hedensjö, MS, is a science reporter and clinical psychologist.

MORE BOOKS *from*
NEW HARBINGER PUBLICATIONS

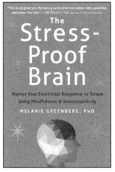
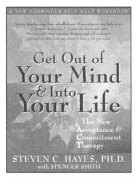
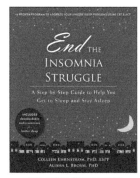
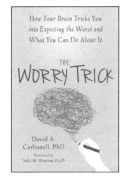
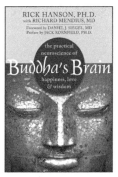
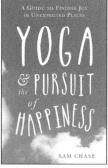
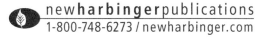

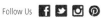

Register your **new harbinger** titles for additional benefits!

When you register your **new harbinger** title—purchased in any format, from any source—you get access to benefits like the following:

- Downloadable accessories like printable worksheets and extra content

- Instructional videos and audio files

- Information about updates, corrections, and new editions

Not every title has accessories, but we're adding new material all the time.

Access free accessories in 3 easy steps:

1. Sign in at NewHarbinger.com (or **register** to create an account).

2. Click on **register a book**. Search for your title and click the **register** button when it appears.

3. Click on the **book cover or title** to go to its details page. Click on **accessories** to view and access files.

That's all there is to it!

If you need help, visit:

NewHarbinger.com/accessories

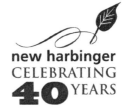

new harbinger
CELEBRATING
40 YEARS